HEART BYPASS SURGERY

YOUR SIMPLY MARVELOUS ROADMAP TO

HEART BYPASS SURGERY

J. Mark Pool, MD

YOUR SIMPLY MARVELOUS ROADMAP TO
HEART BYPASS SURGERY

Paneah Publishing books may be purchased in bulk for educational, business or institutional use. For information, contact

Director of Special Sales
Paneah Publishing
539 W Commerce St
Suite 762
Dallas, TX 75208.

FIRST EDITION

ISBN
hc 979-8-9893676-1-0
pb 979-8-9893676-0-3
e 979-8-9893676-3-4
audio 979-8-9893676-2-7

Printing 10 9 8 7 6 5 4 3 2 1

To the patients and families

I have been blessed to meet,

in the past

and in the future

CONTENTS

FOREWORD

Your Simply Marvelous Roadmap to Heart Bypass Surgery by Dr. J. Mark Pool

It all started in the morning during the summer of 2017. My wife, Millie, who was age 80 at that time, had been walking with a friend around the indoor track at the Cooper Fitness Center in Dallas, Texas. For some unknown reason, she said her arms felt heavy and when she stopped walking those symptoms disappeared.

Concerned, she called me and I encouraged her to come over immediately to our Cooper Clinic for an evaluation. Her resting electrocardiogram was normal so a maximal treadmill stress test was performed. However, within the first few minutes as the heart rate started increasing there were signs of significant abnormality noted on the electrocardiogram but absolutely no chest pain or discomfort. So I terminated the test and immediately called our consultant, invasive cardiologist Dr. Tony Das, and he advised us to "bring her over immediately."

A cardiac catheterization with coronary angiography was performed and revealed multiple vessel disease, too much to be corrected by angioplasty and stent. Only bypass graft surgery would be of value. At that time, Dr. Das said the best and one of the most experienced cardiac bypass surgeons in Dallas, Texas was Dr. John Mark Pool who had done over 3,000 bypass surgical procedures. Unfortunately, he was unavailable to perform the surgery until two days later. Since she was asymptomatic, I asked if I could take her home and bring her back early in the morning the day of the surgery. They said absolutely not! She needed to be hospitalized during the interim since she could have a major coronary event at any time!

Upon reflection, how could my wife of 64 years who had never smoked, was not overweight, and exercised regularly be on the verge of having a major heart attack? That was her question. I was afraid that something else could be responsible for this problem in that she had a known elevation of her serum cholesterol and a high coronary calcification score. For years I had been strongly recommending to Millie that she needed to start taking a statin drug and see if we could stop any progression of the coronary arteriosclerosis.

Sometime later she was asked to speak to a large group of women at an American Heart Association luncheon here in Dallas at which time she told her story. She finished with a strong recommendation to the ladies that "if your physician tells you to do something, do it, even though he might be your husband!"

With that story I am happy to say that the surgery performed by Dr. Pool went well with no complications and she completed a supervised cardiac rehabilitation program. In addition to taking a statin drug (along with coenzyme Q10), she has maintained a good body weight, exercises regularly, and has had no further problems, enjoying life to the fullest!

At the time of this event I don't believe that Dr. Pool had even thought about writing a book entitled "Heart Bypass Surgery," but I am happy he did and I am honored to be writing this foreword.

You will find in this book all the detailed information about heart surgery in general but focusing primarily on coronary artery bypass grafting. For anyone considering heart surgery, this information can help relieve fear and anxiety. I have always believed that knowledge is one the best ways to overcome fear. The first part of the book reveals all the details about how the heart develops and functions so efficiently over a lifetime, never stopping for rest and beating at least 100,000 times every 24 hours without fatigue even in a person of my age of 92.

Remember that the heart starts beating in a child in utero at about 15 weeks and never stops except on rare occasions for a few seconds. This is a miracle of Divine proportion. There is no machine ever made that can function as efficiently for so long as our heart.

In the glossary, Dr. Pool states the heartbeat begins as an electrical impulse originating in the sinoatrial node. Exactly how that occurs is still unclear. I think that both Dr. Pool and I agree that it is most likely Divine intervention since if that heartbeat stops and you are not on a heart-lung bypass machine, all bodily functions will cease in only a few minutes.

The book should be not only of great value to the layman facing heart surgery but should be of great interest to primary care physicians, particularly those interested in cardiology. Not the least, it should be in the curriculum of any medical school, particularly during the freshman year. I truly believe that the book has the potential of saving the lives of innumerable people all over the world and, if so, I know that both Dr. Pool and I would hasten to say, "To God be the glory!"

Kenneth H. Cooper, MD, MPH
Founder & Chairman
Cooper Aerobics | Cooper Clinic

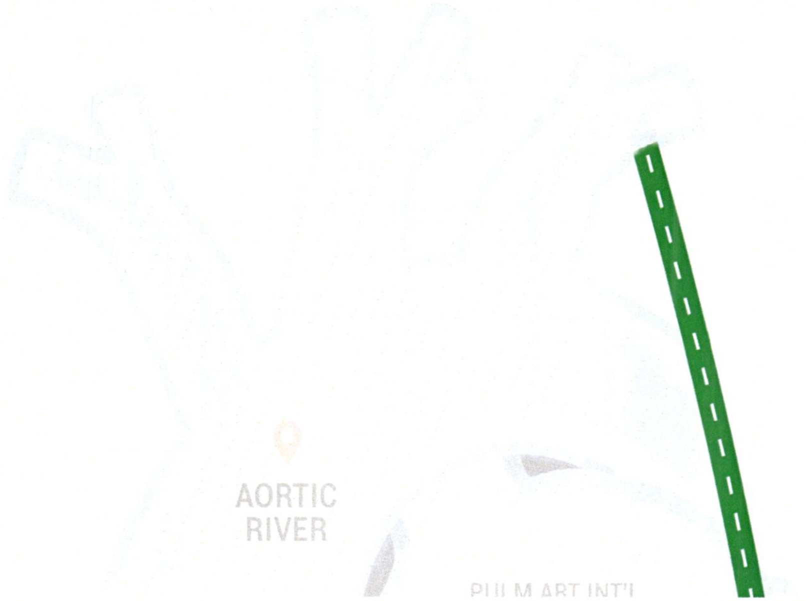

YOUR SIMPLY MARVELOUS ROADMAP TO

HEART BYPASS SURGERY

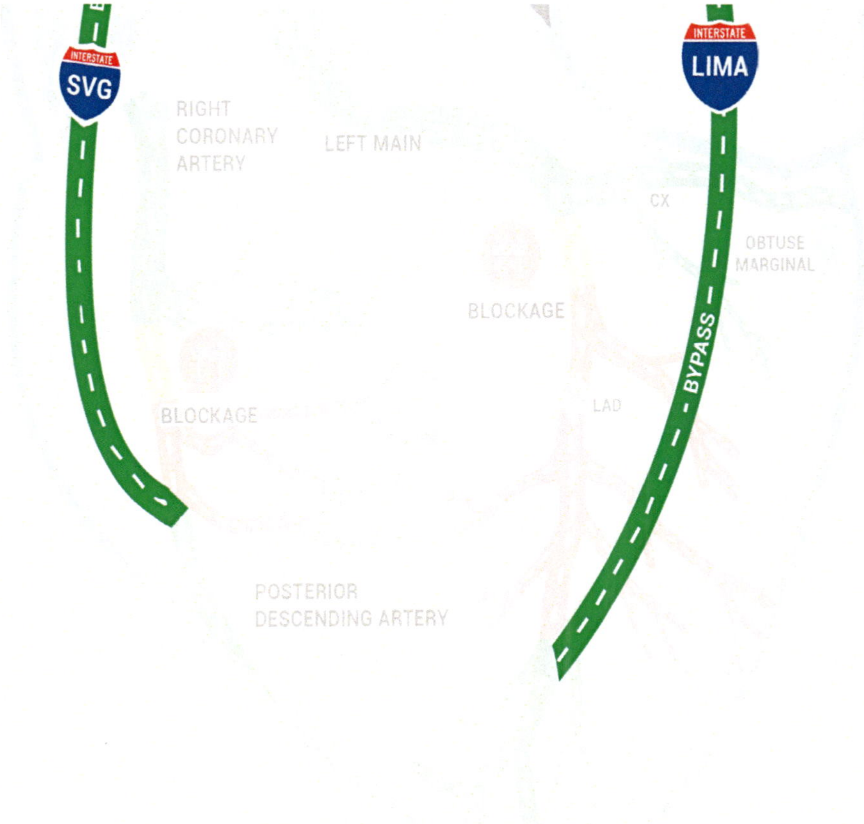

INTRODUCTION

Minor surgery is surgery someone else is having.
When it is yours, surgery is always major.
Anonymous

Heart surgery is a profound thing. That's why I wanted to become a heart surgeon. To do something difficult. Significant.

In the mind of the patient, it is monumental.

Most heart surgery patients only go through it once in a lifetime. Yet most of them would say it is one time too many!

No one wants to have heart surgery, but there are some problems with the heart only surgery can fix, given current technology. And while it is a lot to go through, heart surgery can be life-saving; certainly, it is life-changing.

Reading this book, you likely are facing heart bypass surgery or care for someone who is. Or perhaps you are simply interested to know more about the heart and heart bypass surgery. Whatever your reason, my hope is to provide information and insight to help you in your journey toward better health.

This content is primarily what I want my patients to know in preparing for bypass surgery. I have tried to write it as if I were saying the words to you as we sit together in my office. Although the concepts are serious, I hope the style is light; to wit, if any of my attempts at humor falter, just trust that my tone of voice in person would have made it hilarious. For the record, in case you are wondering by the end of the book, I've got nothing against neurosurgeons or lawyers.

You'll find a few "I think of it" statements in the book. These are not meant to be scientifically valid or factually correct but simply a way to think about a concept, understand, or remember it.

This is not a textbook and there may be errors or inaccurate information; if so, let's blame the editor. Or the publisher. Or the printer… I could go on and on. Surgeons are experts at displacing blame! The displacement skill gets taught from the first day of surgical training.

Please don't take any information here as formal medical advice or a professional recommendation. Always seek the opinion of your personal physician for any specific issue or therapy, and that opinion supersedes any information presented here. If you are my patient and have questions about the content in this book or about your particular situation, of course I will be happy to provide clarification.

There is no doubt more information here than most people need. Or want. If you get bogged down or bored at any point, just skip to the next section. Pick and choose to use this "roadmap" however it may help. Some patients prefer not to know everything about the surgery because details increase their anxiety. Certainly that is not my intent! The details are not meant to slow you down or gross you out but to enhance understanding about your heart, your health, and your heart bypass surgery.

ARE YOU READY?

LET'S TAKE THE FIRST STEP.

START HERE

"If they had just called it 'the stay at home challenge' and posted it on Facebook, the virus would be gone by now."
Anonymous

DO YOU KNOW?

What is the most common disease in the world?
Hint: It is not malaria.

What is the #1 killer of humans?
Hint: It is not cancer.

What is the costliest disease to treat, worldwide?
Hint: It is not COVID-19. (Well, ok, it just might be COVID-19!)

Heart disease is the most common disease in the world, the #1 killer of humans, both men and women, and the costliest disease to treat in terms of worldwide monies spent each year [1]. Heart disease is also the most common cause of death in the USA [2].

It was not always this way. Until around 1900, heart disease was reasonably uncommon in the US, accounting for a minority of deaths [3]. It became more common in the 1920s-1930s and quickly rose to dubious fame as the #1 cause of death.

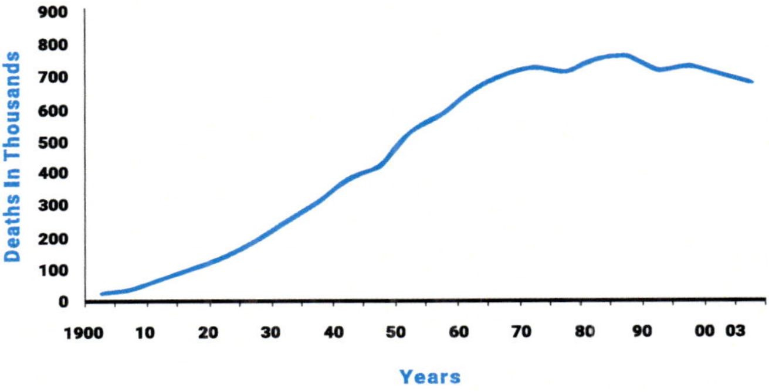

Deaths from diseases of the heart in the USA, 1900-2003 [4]

This was likely due to increased longevity afforded by effective treatment of other life-threatening conditions particularly infectious diseases such as smallpox.

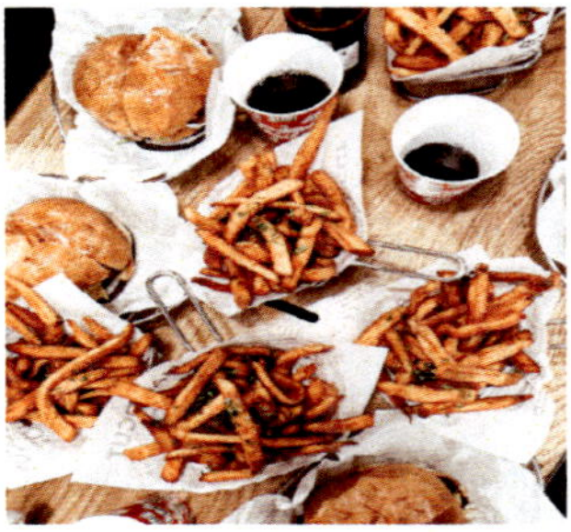

Meanwhile, there have been changes in American diet and daily habits involving overeating and sedentary lifestyle, which have now become ingrained into our culture and passed down from one generation to the next. Interestingly, these American cultural norms have also spread to many other countries across the world.

Currently, over 650,000 Americans die each year from heart disease[2].

The most common form of heart disease is **Coronary Artery Disease** (CAD), where blockages impair blood flow to the heart muscle, which can lead to damage of the muscle. If enough muscle is damaged, delivery of blood to the rest of the body can be impaired.

Though much progress has been made in understanding and treating this disease, there is no known cure. Many of us prefer to live in ignorance or denial, thinking *we* are not susceptible to heart disease.

Have we all just gotten used to the idea of it? You can't really catch CAD from someone else – well, maybe your parents, in a genetic sense. But, you can't catch it like you would a common cold or the flu. Since we can't "catch" it, we don't expend much time or effort defending against it.

By contrast, at the time I am writing this, COVID-19 has taken the lives of over 500,000 Americans in the past year [5]. It certainly is a terrible tragedy, a once-in-a-lifetime pandemic. The global effort and cost to contain this disease can hardly be measured and likely will affect our world for decades.

But astoundingly, heart disease kills more Americans than that *every* year. We've worn masks, stayed 6 feet away from others and taken novel vaccines for COVID-19 – what if we took dramatic steps to change our risk factors for heart disease?

But we haven't acted. We don't act. Not until the problem becomes a crisis. The problem is already severe before we take interest, all too often. It's an intriguing part of our culture that plays out over and over again. Not just in health care but in many areas of life, such as finances, politics and relationships.

Be that as it may, I am willing to bet you are interested in heart disease now more than ever, as you or your loved one are actively wrestling with it.

I am here to help. I cannot *cure* this problem for you — no one can. Not even the dramatic flair of heart bypass surgery will cure it.

But I can help you work toward an effective plan to manage the disease, seeking the highest quality of life and longevity possible, by God's grace.

ARE YOU TALKIN' TO ME?!

Denial is the most predictable of all human responses.
The Architect, Matrix Reloaded [6]

Before getting into the nuts and bolts of heart bypass surgery, let's confront an issue many patients struggle with. It takes the form of the question: Are you sure you have the right patient?!

There are many variations of the idea, which patients have mentioned to me at the time of our consultation:

I never thought this could happen to me.

I thought I was doing all the right things — watching my diet, not smoking, staying active. What was I missing?

This isn't fair — my brother is in a lot worse shape than me and he's never had to have heart surgery! Shouldn't you be talking to him?

What happens if I just go home and don't do anything?

I don't think I can deal with this!

You are likely to experience a flood of emotions when confronted with the need for heart surgery.

I had a patient several years ago who told me it was *unfair* this was happening to him. He was 48 years old at the time, ran 3 miles every day and ate a strict vegetarian diet. But he needed 2 bypasses! He did not seem like someone who would develop heart disease, and he never figured he would have to undergo heart bypass surgery.

I think most people can empathize with his perspective! Many people feel surprised and apprehensive when faced with the need for surgery. Many feel scared. Some patients are shocked. Only a rare few say they "knew this day would come."

I suspect a lot of the negative emotions arise from a sense of the unknown. Patients don't know what to expect, so they expect the worst – and they fear it.

I can relate. I am myself slightly skeptical by nature. I need a good explanation or rationale for things, before I'll go along. The more important the thing, the more explanation I want. Doctors are often good at explaining things, but not always. Patients are usually good at listening, but not always. I have been on both sides. I have had that sense of disbelief in talking with a doctor; I have myself gotten bad news and had trouble taking in the information.

The most dramatic example of this disbelief for me was several years ago:

LETS GET PERSONAL

The morning after my daughter Jane Maddy was born, a pediatrician came into my wife's room. I didn't think much of it since pediatricians see every newborn nowadays. Without introducing himself, he said, "We need to talk about what's wrong." I said, "Excuse me?" He continued, "Yeah, we need to talk about what's wrong with your baby... she is likely to die in the next few days."

What the heck?! I honestly thought he had the wrong room. I thought he didn't know what he was talking about. I had difficulty listening to him because I was still stuck at the first thing he said. But although I didn't fully understand what he was saying, I felt a deep sadness welling up within me.

I know what getting bad news is like. BAD news. News that paralyzes your mind so you can think of nothing else.

Perhaps you feel that needing heart surgery is bad news. Such a feeling is understandable and normal – no one thinks it is wonderful to have a major operation, let alone an operation on the heart. But I encourage my patients to try to focus on the positive: try to focus on the fact that your problem can be helped. You have a problem that requires heart surgery to address, not a problem with no options at all.

I have found that once patients are able to digest the information and come to terms with the challenge they are facing, most are able to move forward with a solid, effective plan. Sometimes, after careful reflection, the plan is to not proceed with surgery. I get that, I respect that; in the end, not having surgery may be the most reasonable option for some patients. Certainly, no patient should be pressured or forced to undergo a therapy he or she does not agree to pursue.

Part of my responsibility as a surgeon is to explain information in a way that helps patients understand their situation and their options, so they can make a decision based on their values and not based on fear or ignorance or external influences. Many times, after having detailed and thoughtful conversations both with me and with their loved ones, patients come to accept surgery as the best option for them, even if they are still not happy with the prospect of going through it.

Is dealing with heart disease and the thought of heart bypass surgery stressful? Invariably.

Life-changing? Certainly.

Something you can ignore? Not indefinitely.

If heart bypass surgery is on your short horizon, you are in good company. Well-known people who have publicly announced they underwent bypass surgery include:

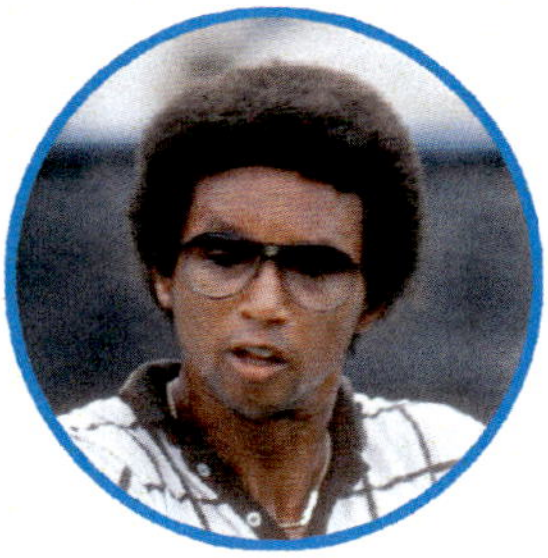

Arthur Ashe [7]
36 years old

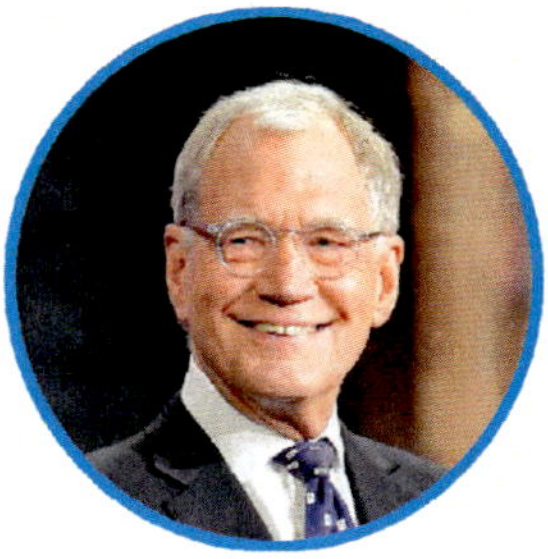

David Letterman [8]
52 years old

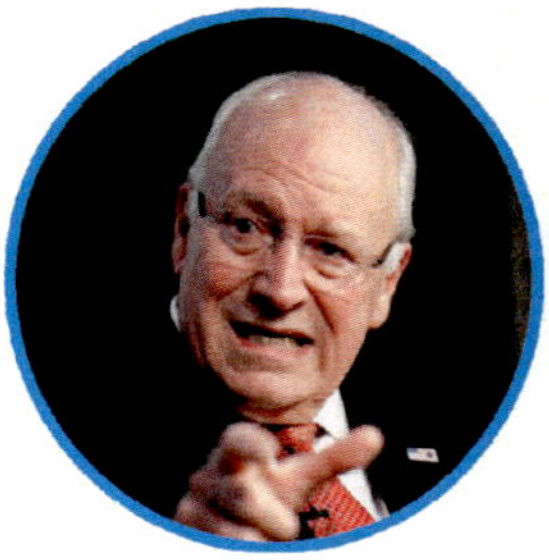

Dick Cheney [9]
47 years old

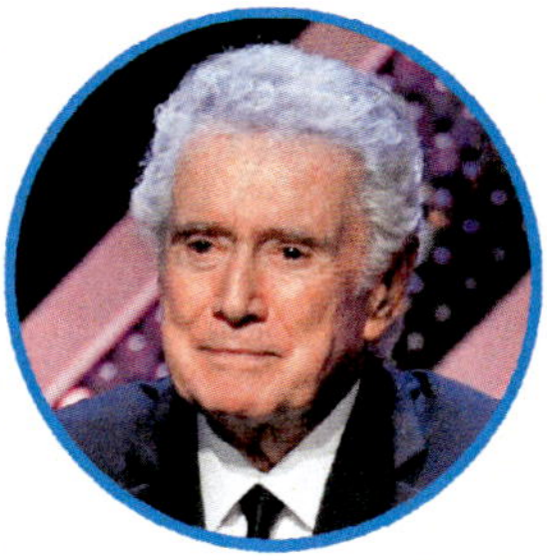

Regis Philbin [10]
74 years old

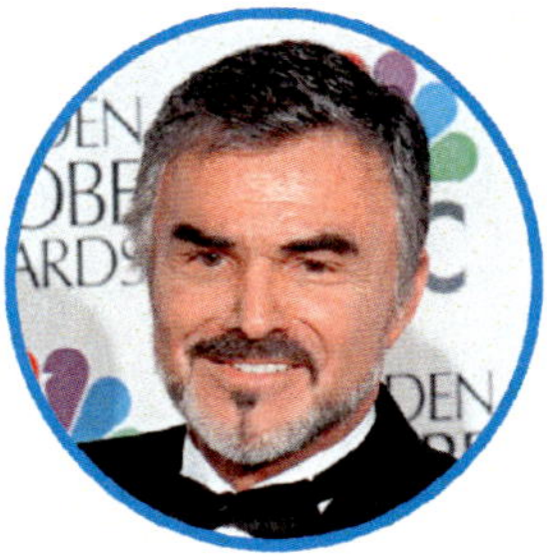

Burt Reynolds [11]
74 years old

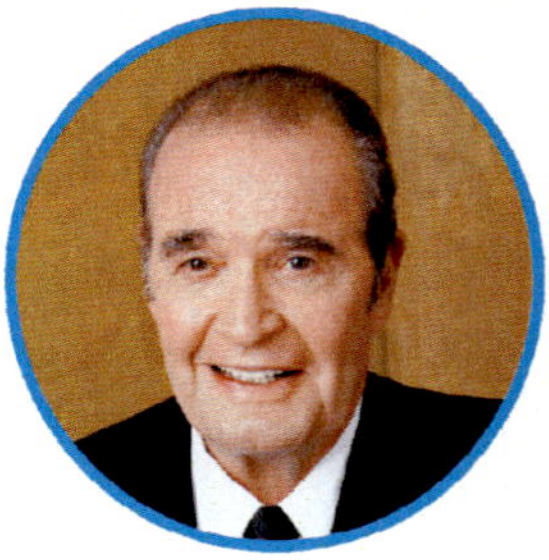

James Garner [12]
60 years old

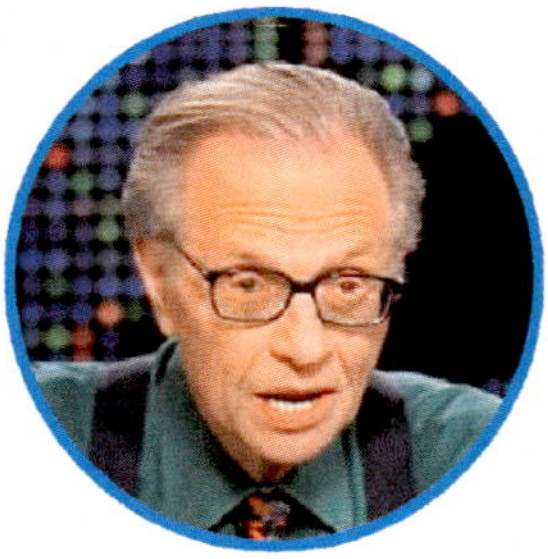

Larry King [13]
53 years old

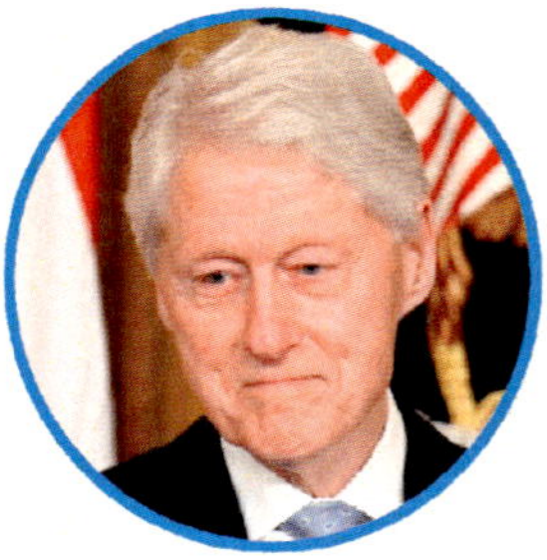

Bill Clinton [14]
58 years old

There are many thousands of other people who have had heart bypass surgery without announcing it publicly. Heart bypass is the most common heart surgery in the US with over 200,000 patients undergoing the operation every year [15].

And I am confident every single one of them had mixed feelings about the situation!

ANATOMY & PHYSIOLOGY FOR THE NON-PHYSICIAN

The search for truth is more precious than its possession.
Albert Einstein [16]

DISCLAIMER

If reading about the scientific details of your predicament does not appeal to you, that is okay. No harm. No foul. No judgment. **Skip to page 95**. Doing so may likely prevent you from tossing this book in the trash can and leaving a 1-star book review on some website. Geeks, nerds, engineers — all my scholastic kinspeople who sensibly leave 5-star book reviews for unnecessarily detailed medical books for lay-people — by all means proceed...

For most of us, the heart is something taken for granted. We take it for granted as long as it's working well, that is. Consider that your heart beats roughly 100,000 times per day. You never have to think about it to make it beat.

From before you were born, to this moment, every moment: lubb-dub, lubb-dub, lubb-dub... When sitting. Walking. Running. Talking. Working. Sleeping. Whatever you are doing, it beats all the time, without *ever* stopping.

Needless to say, if it does stop, there will be a problem!

Interestingly, you couldn't stop it if you wanted to.

You can't make it start, you can't make it stop. How is that? How does the heart function with such reliability and with perpetual independence of your will?

SPECIAL MUSCLE – THE MYOCARDIUM

The heart never stops to rest. It never needs to. The heart muscle is not like any other muscle in your body.

Heart muscle is called **myocardium**. The myocardium has an extremely high metabolic efficiency, allowing myocardial cells to continue to contract even during long periods of high demand. This efficiency is possible because the capillary network in the heart is very dense, the capillaries being where the oxygen moves from the blood into the myocardial cells. There is a 1:1 ratio of capillaries to myocardial cells in the heart [17], meaning that every heart muscle cell has a capillary providing oxygen.

The point is that oxygen is delivered directly to each muscle cell. This direct delivery ensures that given sufficient blood flow, along with oxygen and other nutrients, heart muscle cells – the myocardium – will not fatigue and will not stop contracting because of "overuse."

In addition, the myocardium extracts more oxygen per unit volume of blood than any other tissue of the body [18]. Even at rest, the myocardium extracts roughly 75% of the oxygen in the blood passing through the coronary arteries. By contrast, the kidneys only extract roughly 15% of the oxygen passing through them [19].

DO YOU KNOW?

Where is the darkest blood in the body?
In the coronary sinus, the main vein of the heart itself.

The myocardium extracts the most oxygen from the blood of any organ, resulting in a low oxygen saturation and dark coloration.

In addition to this metabolic efficiency, myocardial cells are linked together in a special way, connected by **intercalated discs**. These connections allow for the transmission of signals between cells and do not exist in any other tissues of the body, only the heart muscle. Charged particles known as ions can easily travel from cell to cell through **gap junctions**, allowing an electrical impulse to move through myocardial cells in a set sequence and almost simultaneously. This close connectivity allows for finely coordinated contractions of the heart as a whole organ.

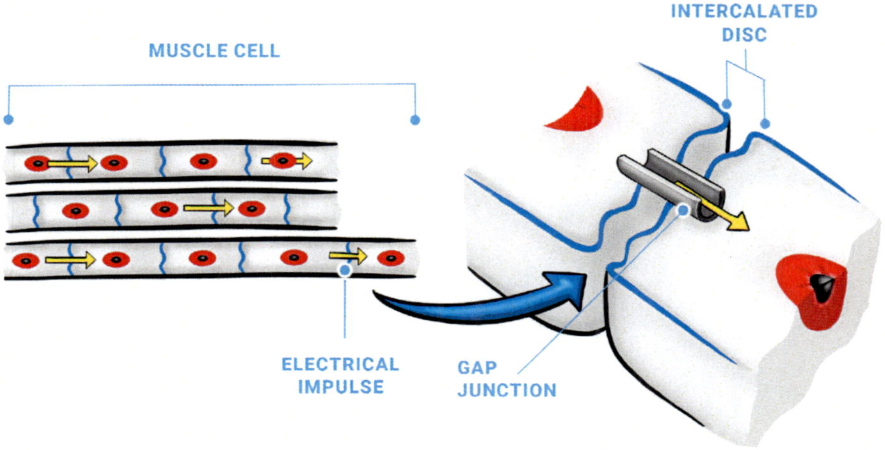

If this coordination is lost, myocardial cells will contract independently and randomly, resulting in a dangerous condition known as **ventricular fibrillation**. Ventricular fibrillation is dangerous because blood is not pumped out of the heart when the myocardial cells contract randomly; rather, the heart writhes like a "bag of worms." The fact that ventricular fibrillation is so rare is a testament to the incredible design of the myocardium.

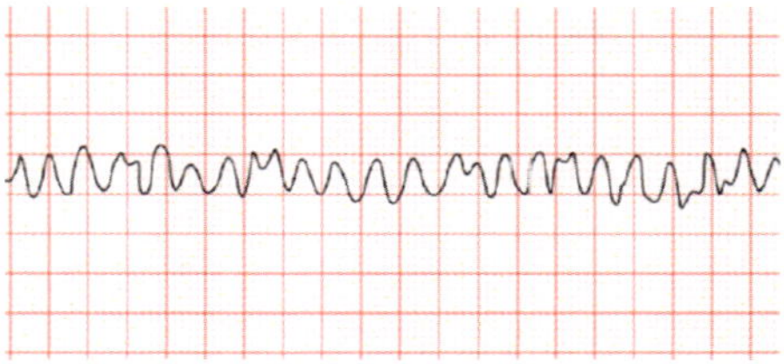

Ventricular fibrillation on EKG

Another interesting aspect of the myocardium is that every myocardial fiber is activated with every heartbeat [17]. Even at rest, even when you are sleeping, every muscle cell in your heart is contracting. Furthermore, every contraction of the myocardium goes to maximal intensity [20]. You can control whether your skeletal muscle contracts weakly or strongly, such as when picking up a feather versus a bowling ball. But each contraction of your heart muscle is maximal, essentially "all or nothing." And, the myocardium never rests or sleeps or takes a break, unlike the activity in your brain, where one area of neurons may be firing while another rests.

A dual threat! The myocardium is super-muscle, the heart a super-organ.

Naturally and logically, this causes heart surgeons to be super-surgeons. Not that I am biased — ahem! (Parenthetically, why do neurosurgeons get all the street cred? The brain isn't so hard to work on — it doesn't move like the heart!).

TAKE HOME POINTS

Myocardial cells are unique in 2 ways:

They contract without ever stopping ==> yet do not fatigue.

They transmit electrical signals ==> yet are not neurons.

The good news is that the myocardium works incredibly well for years on end. The bad news is the human body does not have a way to replace these special cells if damaged or destroyed. The body can regenerate certain portions of liver, bone, skeletal muscle, and skin. But not myocardium.

Shortly after birth, we lose the ability to make new myocardial cells, so if they are damaged and die, they are not replaced. Not even a single myocardial cell can be replaced, let alone many. One myocardial cell dropping out may not affect the strength of the heart in any important way, but many myocardial cells will. If whole sections of myocardial cells are damaged and die, the heart will become weaker and cannot pump blood to the body effectively.

So, take care of your heart! Barring a heart transplantation, your heart is the only one you get. Literally — at the cellular level.

Research is being done in this area. Adult zebrafish can regenerate myocardial cells [21], as can some amphibians (frogs). These organisms are being studied to determine how their

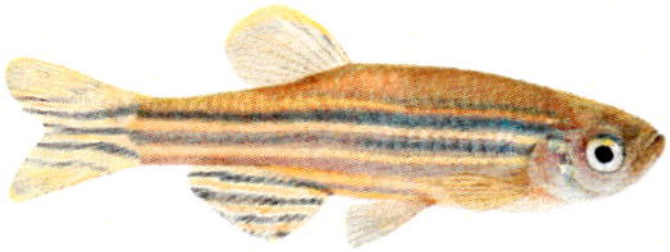

myocardial cells are replaced. Stem cells may be the answer but not much is understood about how to harness the power of stem cells for this purpose. Such therapies certainly are nowhere near ready for primetime use in humans.

But who knows? Maybe some years from now, stents and bypass surgery will not be needed, because stem cells can be used to grow more myocardium if damage occurs.

TAKE HOME POINTS

Myocardial cells CANNOT be replaced.

CIRCULATION

Since ancient times, it has been known that the heart is crucial to life. But not every organism has a heart. *Some* lawyers do, but it is often difficult to tell without invasive testing. Other than lawyers, the largest animal without a heart is the jellyfish; a jellyfish does not have a heart and does not have any blood. Starfish and sea cucumbers also do not have hearts. These organisms receive oxygen directly into their tissues from the water in which they live.

DO YOU KNOW?

Does any animal have more than one heart?
Yes! An octopus has 3 hearts. So does a squid. The hagfish has 4 hearts.

It is said that an earthworm has 5 hearts but an earthworm "heart" is only a special tube, not a complex multi-chambered organ.

Oxygen will only move — the fancy term is **diffuse** — directly into cells over a short distance, so larger and more complex organisms use blood to carry oxygen to tissues. The blood is pumped by the heart.

Humans have a single 4-chambered heart, as do all mammals and birds. Most reptiles and amphibians have a 3-chambered heart, while fish have a 2-chambered heart.

The chambers of the heart are hollow with walls made up of myocardial cells, which squeeze, or contract. Many myocardial cells contracting in coordination reduces the size of the chamber, thereby moving blood out and allowing the heart to function as a pump.

A pump moves fluid, usually from an area of low pressure to an area of higher pressure. For humans, and in fact all mammals, the heart is essentially two pumps in one.

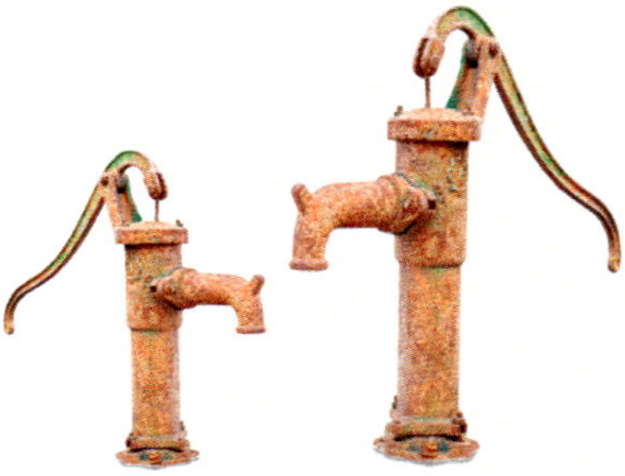

The right pump sends blood to the lungs and the left pump sends blood to the body. The two pumps come packaged together at birth as the right and left sides of the heart.

The right pump — consisting of the right atrium and right ventricle — sends blood to the lungs and then back to the heart in a pathway called the **pulmonary circulation**.

The left pump — consisting of the left atrium and left ventricle — sends blood to the body and then back to the heart in a pathway called the **systemic circulation**.

In a normal adult heart, there is no direct connection for blood to flow between the two sides of the heart.

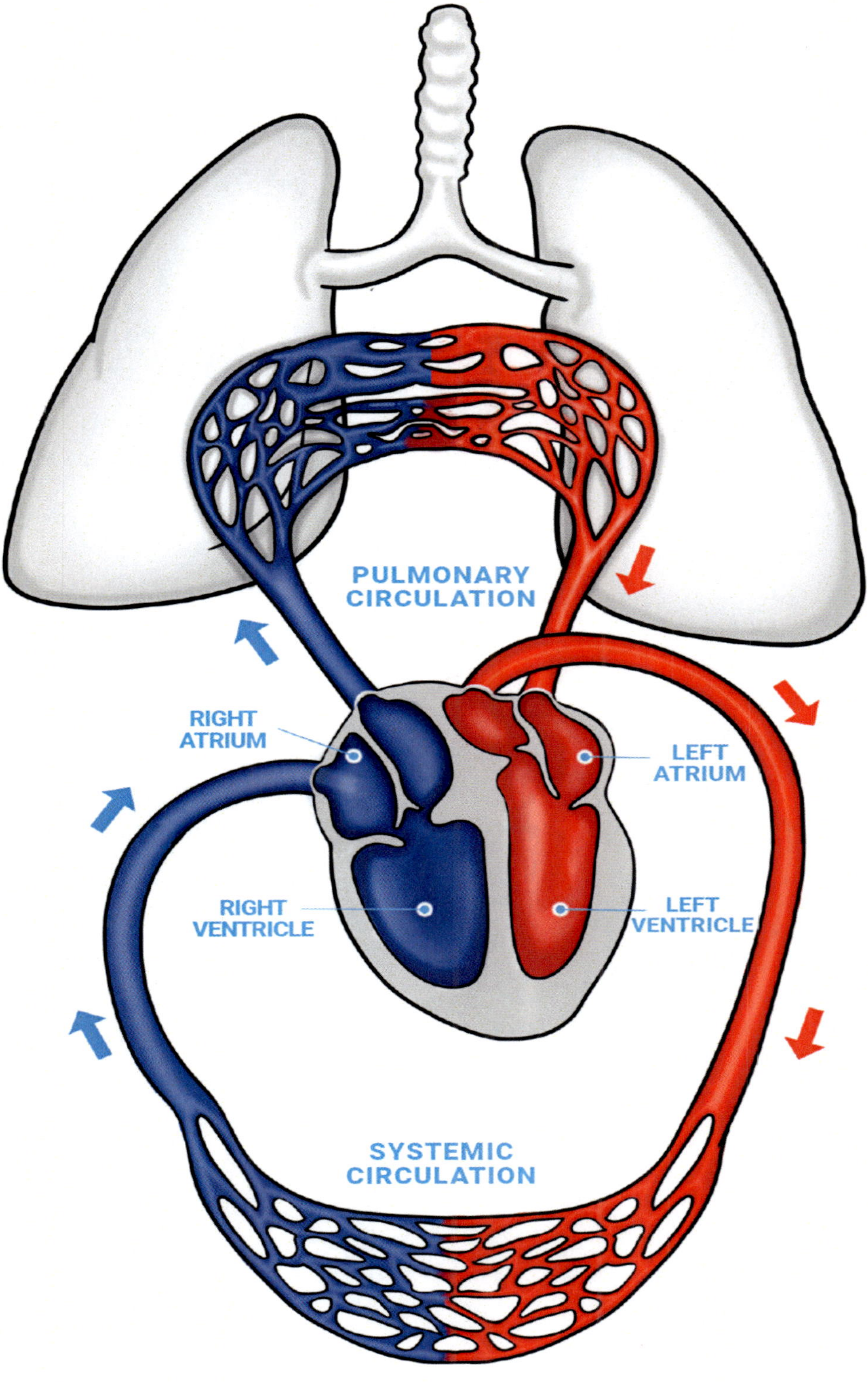
PULMONARY
CIRCULATION
RIGHT
ATRIUM
LEFT
ATRIUM
RIGHT
VENTRICLE
LEFT
VENTRICLE
SYSTEMIC
CIRCULATION

The lung arteries – aka the **pulmonary arteries** – have a blood pressure that is low such that the right pump does not have to produce much work; thus, the right ventricle (RV) is not thick and not as strong as the left ventricle (LV). Usually, the mass of the RV is around 1⁄6 that of the LV [21]. The left ventricle is normally fairly thick since it creates the blood pressure of the arteries of the body (your new friend, the systemic circulation), which is much higher than the blood pressure in the lungs.

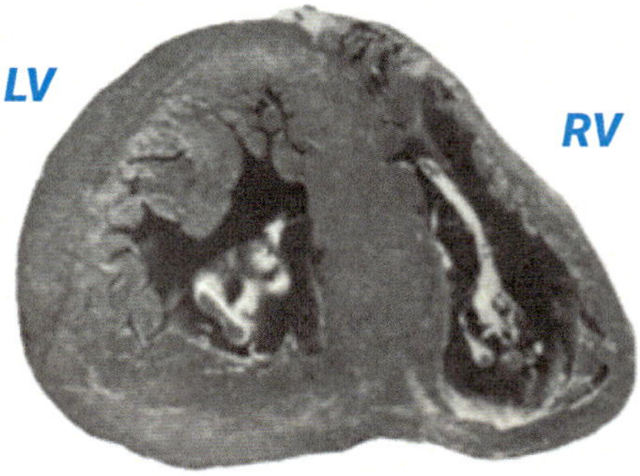

Sectioned ventricles, viewed toward the apex [22]

If the blood pressure in the lungs or the body becomes very high, extra work is required of the ventricles to move the blood. If this extra work continues over an extended period of time, the walls of the ventricles become thicker. Such an increase in the thickness of the walls is called **hypertrophy**.

A normal pressure in the lung arteries is 20/10 mmHg or so, whereas a normal pressure may be 120 /80 mmHg in the systemic arteries.

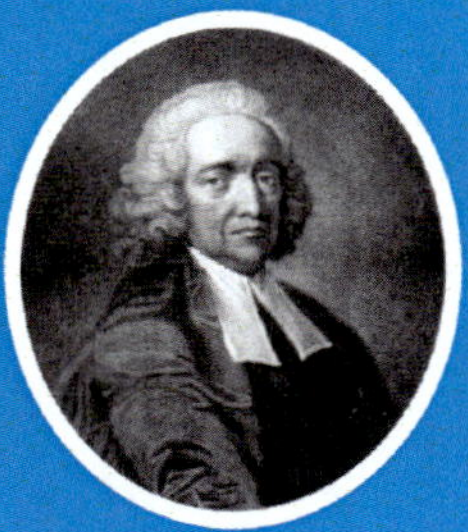

COULD YOU DO THAT?

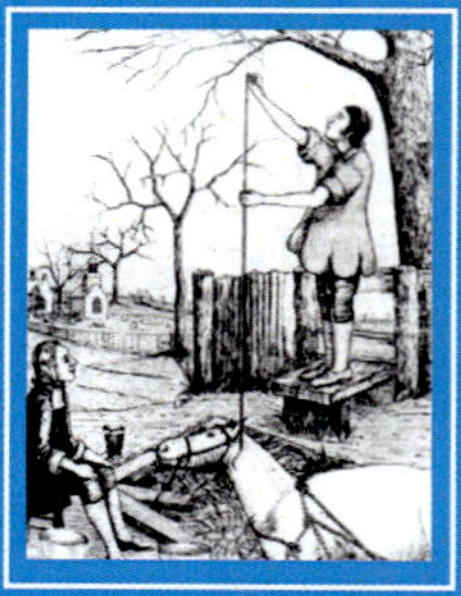

Stephen Hales was the first person to measure blood pressure. An English clergyman, the Reverend had a range of interests, including how the human body works. In **1727**, he placed a glass tube into the femoral artery of a horse, and the **column of blood** rose to nearly **9 feet.**

Note, the artist's depiction incorrectly shows access to the horse's carotid artery in the neck rather than the femoral artery in the groin [23].

Although they may sound similar, the terms systolic and systemic have very different meanings. I think of it as systemic relates to the whole system of blood vessels in the body, while systolic sounds like how "tall" the blood pressure column rises.

Blood pressure consistently higher than normal is called **hypertension**; non-medical people often call it "high blood pressure." Hypertension is a major risk factor for disease and disability, affecting millions of people.

The ventricular chambers are roughly shaped like a cone, with muscle making up the sides. When the muscle cells contract and shorten, the volume of each chamber decreases and the pressure increases, moving blood out. The blood follows the path of least resistance and could possibly move right back where it came from, so heart valves open and close in a specific way to be sure the blood moves only one direction.

EXTRA CREDIT

The shape of the ventricle relates to the pressure it must create. A more **elliptical shape** is needed for **higher pressures**.

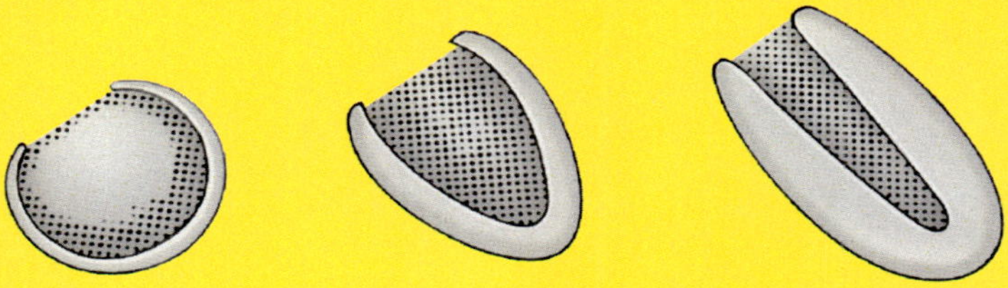

Blood pressure:	FROG 30 mmHg	HUMAN 120 mmHg	GIRAFFE 300 mmHg

Figure adapted from [24]

When a human heart becomes severely weak, the walls bulge out and give it a ball-like or globular shape, much like the shape of the lower-pressure heart of the frog.

There is a spiral orientation of many of the myocardial fibers, such that the heart twists slightly to the right when it contracts.

Blood comes into the heart through veins, namely the **inferior vena cava** from below and the **superior vena cava** from above. I think of it as superior is the best or on top, much like a book about heart surgery is superior to a book about neurosurgery. These two mega-veins drain blood into the **right atrium**.

The blood then moves from the right atrium through the tricuspid valve into the **right ventricle**. The right ventricle pumps the blood through the **pulmonic valve** into the pulmonary arteries, which branch many times, eventually becoming microscopic in size. The microscopic arteries "turn into" **arterioles**, which can expand and contract to control the amount of blood flowing through them. The arterioles give rise to **capillaries**.

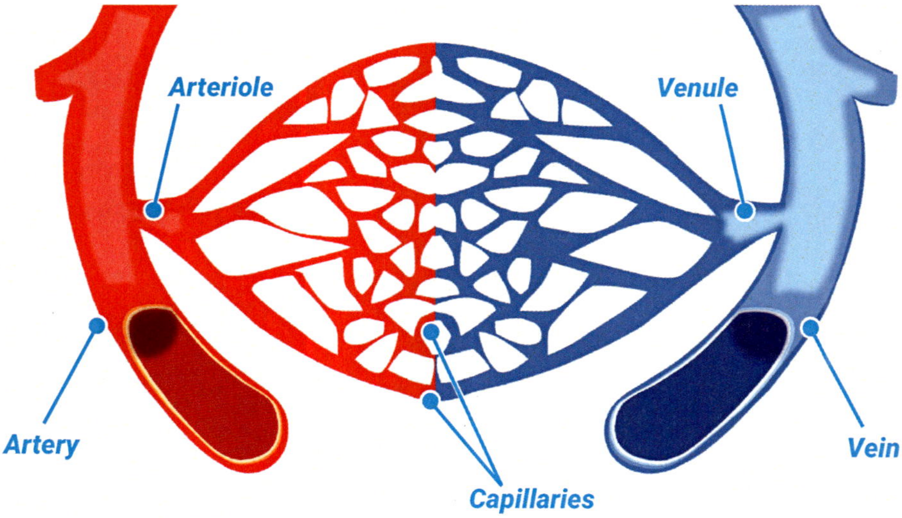

Capillaries are microscopic and form the smallest channels in the circulatory system — it would take 10 capillaries to add up to the width of a human hair. Red blood cells move single-file through capillaries. At this microscopic level, oxygen from the atmosphere moves from the **air sacs** of the lungs into the blood, and carbon dioxide moves out of the blood and into the air sacs to be breathed out.

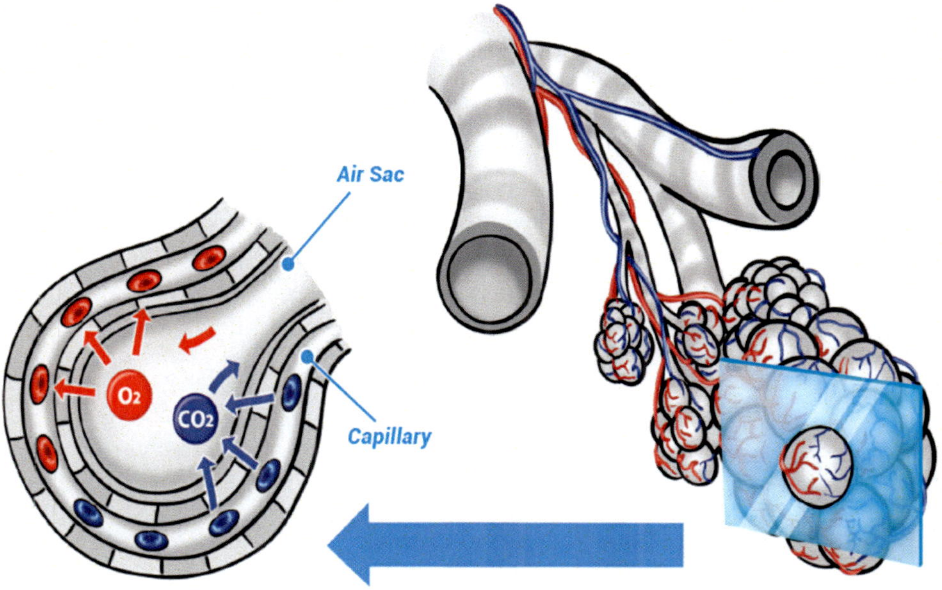

DO YOU KNOW?

How many air sacs are present in your lungs?
700,000,000! [25]

If spread out one layer thick, the air sacs in your lungs would cover half a tennis court [26].

The blood — now with a lot of oxygen in it — moves through **venules**, which can also expand and contract to control the amount of blood moving through them. The venules give rise to veins, which become larger and larger, carrying blood back to the heart and into the **left atrium**.

The blood then moves through the **mitral valve** and into the **left ventricle**. The left ventricle is the strongest part of the heart and pumps the blood through the **aortic valve** into the **aorta**. The aorta is the biggest blood vessel in the body, about the size of a garden hose; it carries blood to the organs of the body, dividing into smaller and smaller arteries along the way. Arterioles are next in line and then capillaries, where oxygen is delivered within the tissues.

Blood returns to the heart through venules and then veins, carrying carbon dioxide, a waste product of cells. Meanwhile, nutrients from food are picked up by blood in the intestines while toxins are filtered out of the blood by the kidneys and liver.

A complex system, to be sure! Another amazing thing we too often take for granted.

DO YOU KNOW?

How long does it take for blood to make a complete circuit through the circulation?
About 60 seconds in a human, at a heart rate of 60 beats per minute.

The time for completion of the circulation varies depending on the size of an animal. It takes around 10 seconds for a mouse, which has an average HR of 600 bpm, versus 2 minutes for an elephant, which has an average HR of 30 bpm. It consistently takes about 60 heart-beats no matter the size of the organism [18].

Most adults have roughly 5 liters or $1\frac{1}{2}$ gallons of blood, which the heart pumps every minute. About 60% of the blood is present in the veins at any given time, while 10% is inside the heart and 10% in the lungs. About 20% of the blood is in the arteries [27]. I would have guessed the blood is divided evenly $^{50}/_{50}$ between the arteries and veins, but it's not!

TAKE HOME POINTS

The right atrium & ventricle move blood through the pulmonary circulation, where oxygen is picked up.

The left atrium & ventricle move blood through the systemic circulation, where oxygen is delivered.

Congratulations! You now know more about the circulation than every person who lived until 1628!

Dr. William Harvey figured out the basics of the circulation and published his findings in ***De Motu Cordis*** in 1628. Some people have described this book as the most important book in the history of medicine, because this one book changed how people understood the body, blood, and the heart.

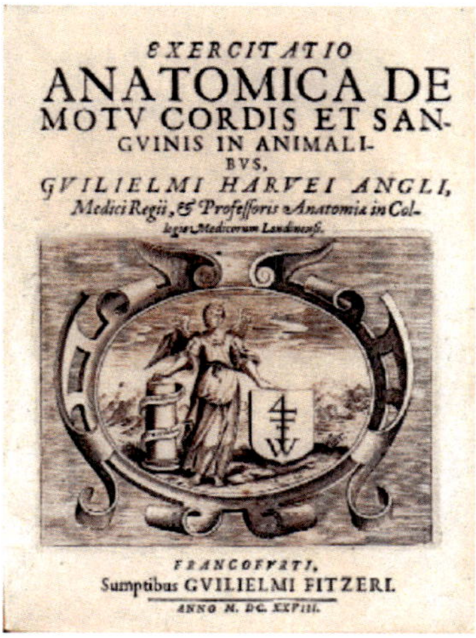
EXERCITATIO
ANATOMICA DE
MOTV CORDIS ET SAN-
GVINIS IN ANIMALI-
BVS,
GVILIELMI HARVEI ANGLI,
Medici Regii, & Professoris Anatomiæ in Col-
legio Medicorum Londinensi.

FRANCOFVRTI,
Sumptibus GVILIELMI FITZERI.
ANNO M. DC. XXVIII.

Title page of De Motu Cordis [28]

Dr. Harvey's book broke the intellectual stranglehold of earlier ideas, opening the door to further scientific progress in the field of medicine. Scientists began to think about and question and explore the body, rather than blindly accept traditional teachings.

For well over 1,000 years, the teachings of a man known as Galen of Pergamon had been taken as scientific fact. Among other things, Galen taught that venous blood was made in the liver and moved through veins to tissues, where it was consumed.

He also taught that arterial blood was made in the heart and moved through arteries to tissues, where it was consumed. The tissues consumed a lot of blood according to Galen!

After Dr. Harvey's breakthrough and the hundreds of years of scientific progress since, we now know that blood is made by your bone marrow, blood moves through veins away from tissues, and the heart pumps blood through arteries to the body tissues and then to veins and back to the heart through a never-ending circuit.

Blood is never "consumed" as Galen would have described it, but damaged blood cells are removed by the spleen and liver.

DO YOU KNOW?

How many blood cells does your bone marrow make each day?
About 500 billion!

About 500 billion blood cells are also destroyed each day.

Not all human bones have marrow. Marrow is mostly found in ribs, the sternum, vertebrae and bones of the pelvis.

It is commonly said that an adult's heart is roughly the size of a fist, but it is really more the size of two fists. A man's heart usually weighs around 10 oz — slightly less than a can of soda; a woman's heart usually weighs slightly less. Either way it's a small size for such an important organ!

DO YOU KNOW?

What organ of the human body weighs the most?
The skin!

Skin is the heaviest organ, weighing 8-10 lbs for most people. Of internal organs, the liver is heaviest, weighing 4-5 lbs, the brain weighs 3-4 lbs, and each lung weighs 2-3 lbs.

The heart is located in the middle of the chest between the lungs, positioned slightly toward the left side.

There is a 3rd circulation, believe it or not — the **coronary circulation**. The coronary circulation carries blood to the heart itself and back again.

SIGNALS

The heart is primarily muscle and connective tissue; the muscle contracts to move blood and the connective tissue holds the muscle together. How does muscle and connective tissue know when to contract? And how does the rate of contraction change, being low when you sleep and high when you exercise, for instance? How does it do that?

There is no nerve to the heart; or at least, there is not a single nerve to the heart. Not a large nerve you could find in Anatomy Lab or that a heart surgeon must be careful to avoid cutting during surgery.

Most muscles in the body have one specific nerve which controls it — that is, most *voluntary* muscles do, muscles you decide to contract or relax. If the nerve is cut, the muscle will not contract anymore. But as you know, the heart is not composed of voluntary muscle — it is composed of myocardium.

You cannot consciously control the contraction of your heart, as you might control the muscles in your arms or legs. It may be possible to adjust the heart rate some through meditation or concentration, but in general, you cannot consciously cause your heart to start or stop when you want, specifically on cue.

While there is no large, single nerve to the heart, there are fibers of nerves which help control the heart and also provide feedback from the heart to other body systems.

One such nerve is the **vagus nerve**, pronounced "VAY-gus." The vagus nerve provides input to the heart, lungs and digestive system, as well as muscles in the throat and your vocal cords. Vagus comes from a Latin word that means wandering, the same root word that gives us the words vagabond and vague. The vagus nerve has branches that "wander" around the chest and torso.

The vagus nerve is part of the **Autonomic Nervous System** (ANS), which **auto**matically controls your body without you having to think about it. Breathing, heart rate, digestion, and many other functions of your body are governed by this system.

The ANS has a **sympathetic** portion and a **parasympathetic** portion, which basically balance each other. The vagus nerve is part of the parasympathetic system.

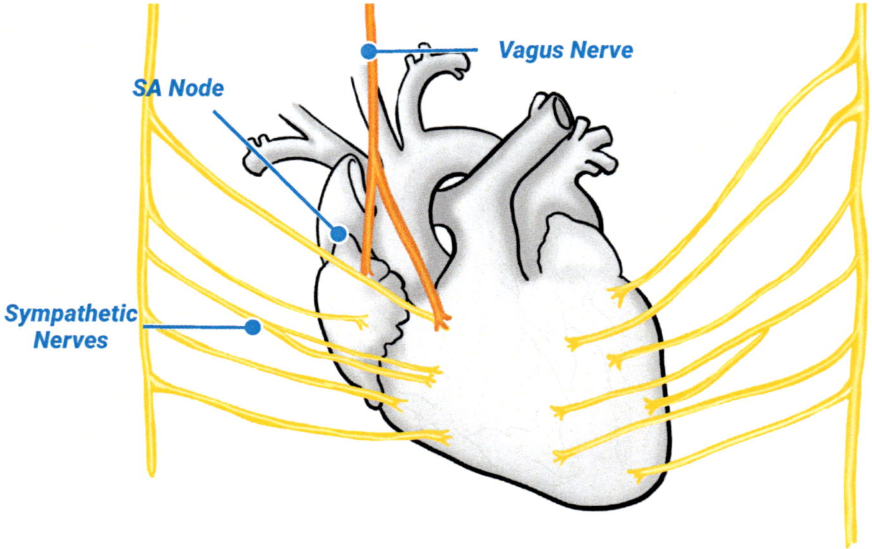

Activation of the vagus nerve lowers the heart rate, like the brake slows the speed of your car. I think of it as pa***R***asympathetic = b**R**ake to slow down and ***R***elax in Vegas.

There are also fibers to the heart from the sympathetic portion of the ANS. The sympathetic system helps control the body's involuntary response to stressful situations, often called "**fight or flight**."

Your heart rate will almost immediately go up if you are surprised by a threat: when you hear hissing and see a forked tongue, your body reacts, faster than you can consciously realize the menace is a lawyer. The sympathetic system acts like the body's accelerator. I think of it as ***S***ympathetic = fight the **S**nakes or run away fa***S***t!

TAKE HOME POINTS

The autonomic nervous system automatically controls your body:

PaRasympathetic => Relax in vagus = bRake, slows the heart

Sympathetic => fight the Snakes = accelerate, Speeds the heart

So the vagus nerve with its parasympathetic fibers slows your heart and sympathetic fibers speed it up. Sadly, with competing signals, the heart won't know what to do if you see a lawyer while in Vegas, leaving you highly vulnerable to a rhetorical attack.

But your heart will continue to beat even if all nerve fibers to it are severed. Really? Yes! Once again, most muscles of the body won't function if the nerve is cut. But the myocardium is special: even with no nerves at all — such as after a heart transplant — it will still beat.

How can that be?

SA NODE

The heart can beat without input from *any* nerves. Or input from any other tissues of the body for that matter. There are special cells in your heart which create electricity. It is the electrical signals which cause the heart muscle cells to contract, thereby causing the heart to beat.

(Purists may insist that strictly speaking the signals are not *electrical* since they do not involve the movement of electrons; rather, the signals involve movement of charged molecules called **ions** across cell membranes — but I think of it like purists are welcome to write their own book!)

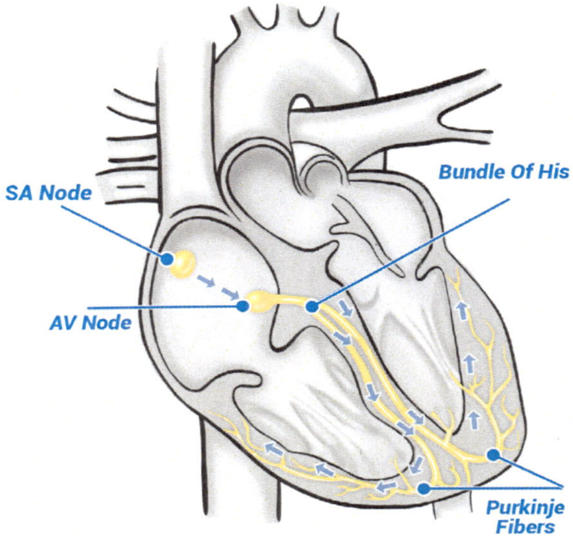

These special cells are found in the **SA node,** which is short for SinoAtrial node. The SA node exists near a sinus, or recessed area, close to the superior vena cava as it empties into the right atrium. These special cells create an electrical signal which moves through the atrial wall to the **AV node**, located near the junction of the atria and ventricles.

While most of the heart is composed of myocardium, which can transmit electrical impulses (remember the intercalating discs?), the connective tissue between the atria and the ventricles does not conduct. The connective tissue is insulating and electrical impulses cannot pass through it, so electrical signals cannot get from the atria to the ventricles.

Except for one pathway — the AV node. The AV node is made of special cells that conduct electricity. The AV node is the only way to get from the atria to the ventricles, electrically speaking.

The electrical signal from the SA node is conducted through and amplified by the AV node. It is then transmitted to the ventricles, through a specialized pathway called the **Bundle of His**.

The Bundle of His has left and right bundles, which travel down the ventricles and give rise to **Purkinje fibers**; these fibers transmit the signal to ventricular myocardial cells, thereby causing contraction.

The myocardial cells then re-set electrically as they relax, getting ready for the next electrical signal and next contraction.

Without input from nerves, the SA node will usually fire an electrical impulse 60-100 times per minute. When the conduction system is working normally, this consistent firing results in a **normal sinus rhythm**, which is steady, like a metronome.

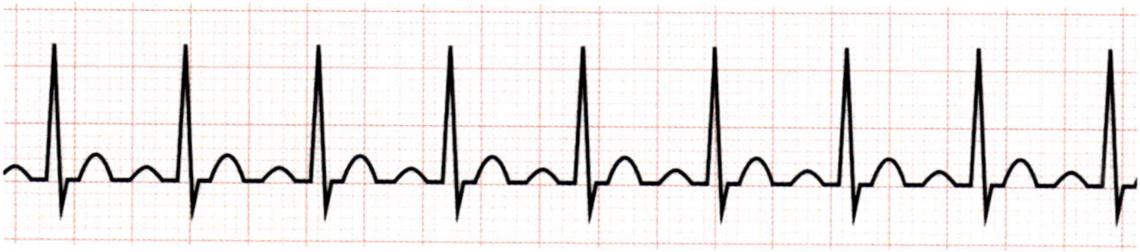

Normal sinus rhythm on EKG

Fibers from the vagus nerve and sympathetic nervous system can adjust the firing rate of the SA node. If a problem with the SA node develops, or at any point along the conduction system, **a cardiac dysrhythmia** may develop.

Dysrhythmia is a fancy medical term for abnormal rhythm. Instead of being nice and steady, a dysrhythmia involves irregularity of the beat. A common cardiac dysrhythmia affecting bypass patients is **atrial fibrillation** (afib), which is discussed on page 118.

In addition to input from nerves, the SA node is also affected by hormones. And not just the SA node — many cells in the heart are affected by hormones.

HORMONAL INFLUENCE

The heart is affected by many chemicals circulating in the blood. A chemical produced in one area of the body which acts as a signal on a tissue or organ elsewhere in the body is called a **hormone**. Hormones are generally made in glands.

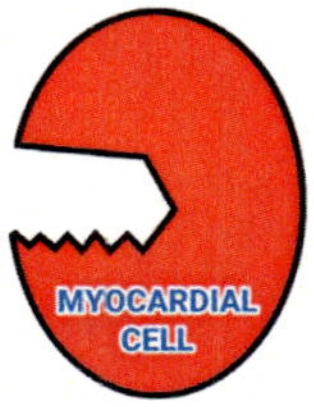

UNSTIMULATED

Adrenaline is an important hormone; it is also known as epinephrine. Adrenaline is made mostly in the adrenal glands and has some effect on almost every tissue of the body. It acts upon specific **receptors** on many types of cells. I think of receptors like keyholes for cells, where the surface of the cell has a shape which fits the hormone.

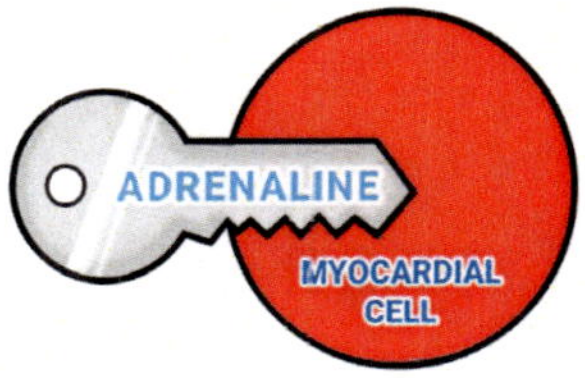

STIMULATED

The hormone is the key — the medical term is **agonist** — which fits into the receptor; the combination of the two unlocks a certain response by the cell. Different types of cells have different receptors; thus, hormones can act on one cell and not the cell next to it. Consequently, hormones have different actions on different parts of the body.

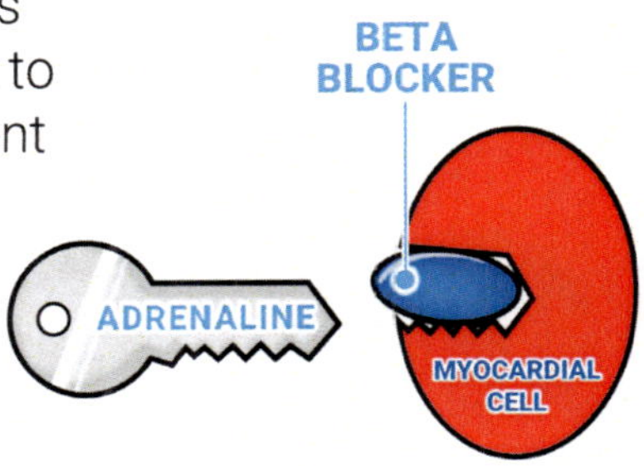

UNSTIMULATED

Some cells have a so-called Beta receptor, which fits the shape of adrenaline . When adrenaline binds to Beta receptors of the SA node cells, the heart rate increases, because adrenaline changes the SA node cells in a way that speeds up the firing of electrical signals by the SA node.

In addition, myocardial cells have Beta receptors, and the muscle contracts more vigorously when adrenaline binds the receptors.

Medications known as **Beta-blockers** bind to the Beta receptors and block them so that adrenaline cannot fit into the keyhole anymore. Without adrenaline binding the cells, the SA node is less stimulated so the heart rate goes down; likewise, myocardial cells are less stimulated to contract so the blood pressure goes down.

There are additional hormones such as insulin, thyroid hormone, cortisol, growth hormone and many others which help regulate the heart rate.

TAKE HOME POINTS

Electrical signals are created by the SA node, pass through the AV node & cause myocardial cells to contract.

The vagus nerve slows down & sympathetic nerve fibers speed up the SA node.

Numerous hormones such as adrenaline have effects on the SA node, which medications can block.

Although the heart has the ability to beat without input from nerves or hormones, the normal regulation of the heart rate involves all of these factors and is quite complicated!

EKG

As you now know, my non-purist friend, the heart runs on electricity; that is, electrical impulses cause the myocardial cells to contract, and their coordinated contraction moves blood. Fortunately, the electrical activity of the heart can be measured and recorded, helping us better understand the heart.

A tracing of the electrical potentials of the heart is called an **electrocardiogram**, or ECG. In a general sense, the ECG shows the movement of the electrical signal from the SA node through the AV node and into the ventricles.

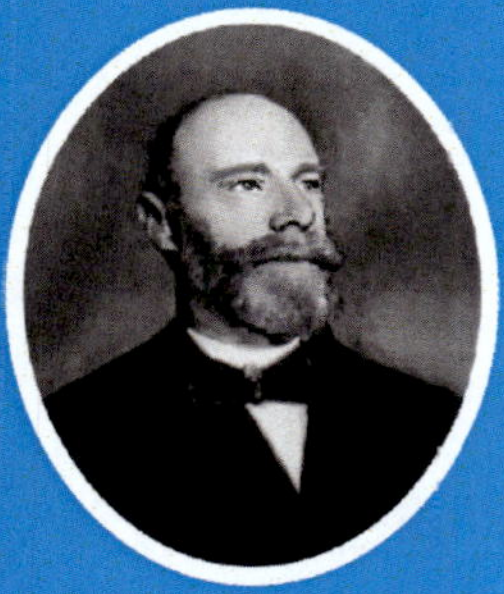

COULD YOU DO THAT?

Dr. Willem Einthoven, a Dutch physiologist, invented the first **practical EKG machine** in **1895** and won the Nobel prize for it in 1924.

We take it for granted now, but when it was invented, the EKG machine was probably the **most sophisticated scientific instrument in existence** [29].

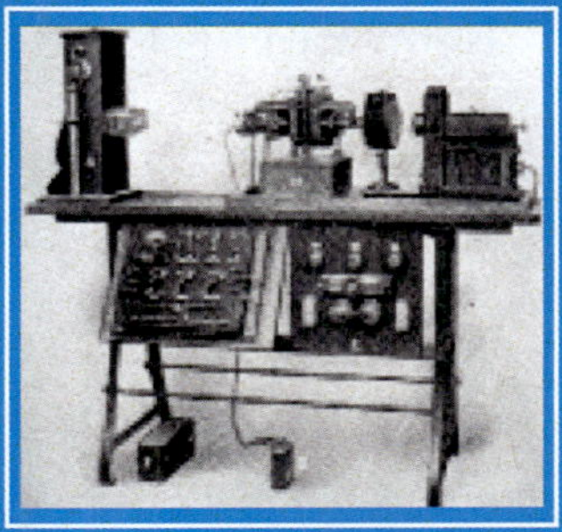

Early Einthoven EKG machine [30]

An ECG is also known as an **EKG**. EKG comes from the original German spelling **e**lektro**k**ardio**g**ramm, a term coined by Dr. Einthoven, inventor of the EKG machine. His first EKG machine weighed over 500lbs and required five people to operate it. Knowing this may help you appreciate the small, portable machine we currently use!

Dr. Einthoven used the letters P, Q, R, S, T to describe major points of deflection.

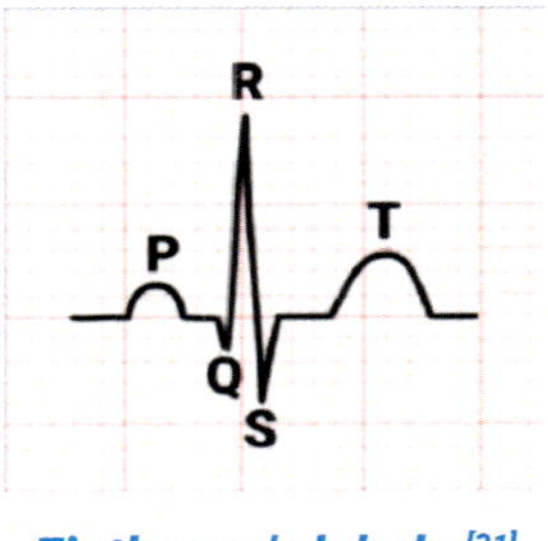

Einthoven's labels [31]

In modern use, several leads from the EKG machine are placed on the patient's chest using adhesive, and machine senses changes in electrical potentials between the leads, providing a tracing which can be interpreted by a healthcare provider. An EKG is not invasive and does not cause pain, other than mild discomfort when the adhesive is removed. Electricity does NOT flow from the machine into the patient, so there is no need to fear an electric shock.

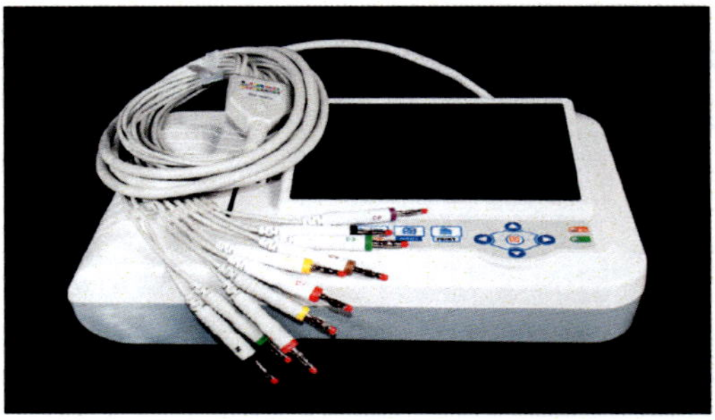

Modern EKG machine

An EKG provides information about the heart rate and rhythm. It can also show subtle information about the size of the heart and sometimes can show evidence of a heart attack.

As a patient, it is important to know that an EKG does not show **CAD** (coronary artery disease), blockages in the arteries of the heart. An EKG might show evidence of a complication of CAD, such as evidence of a heart attack or an enlarged heart, but an EKG is not a good test for detecting CAD.

Many patients have told me they assumed their heart was "fine" because they had a normal EKG, only to find out later they have CAD. If there is suspicion of CAD, a stress test is a better screening test rather than an EKG alone (even a stress test can miss CAD, though).

An EKG is good for showing evidence of a particular type of heart attack called STEMI. Because of this, an EKG is a standard part of the evaluation of any patient with chest pain.

HEART ATTACK

A "heart attack" occurs when blood flow is interrupted to the heart muscle and the muscle is damaged; the medical term is **myocardial infarction**. When cells do not have enough blood flow but damage hasn't happened yet, the term **ischemia** is used. The longer heart muscle cells are ischemic, the more likely infarction — cell death — will occur.

There are two main types of heart attacks: **STEMI** and **NSTEMI**.

STEMI stands for **ST E**levation **M**yocardial **I**nfarction and is pronounced "STEM-ee." A STEMI is a type of heart attack that makes the ST segments appear higher, or elevated, on an EKG compared to normal.

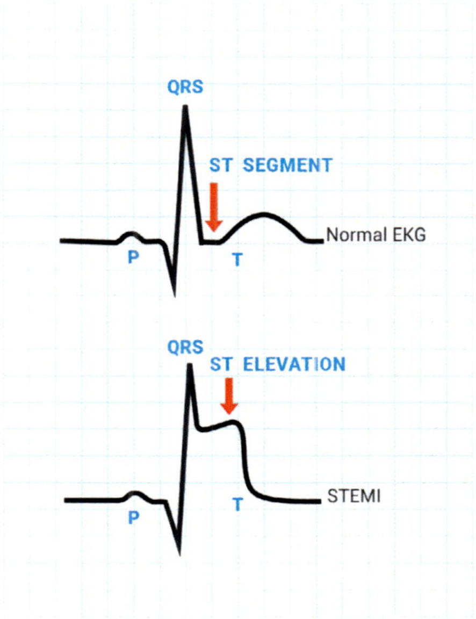

This happens because the myocardial cells do not get enough oxygen and the movement of electricity (ok, ok... ions; enough with the hate, purists!) doesn't flow in a normal way.

What typically happens with a STEMI is a **plaque** ruptures in one of the arteries of the heart. Plaque is a build-up of fats and cholesterol, as well as a nano-particle of every twinkie and doughnut you ever ate.

The plaque builds-up with a smooth surface, but this can become disrupted, exposing proteins to the blood which had been hidden within the plaque. Why a plaque ruptures at a given moment — the exact trigger, why it happened that day at that time — is not well-understood.

The interesting thing is the plaque rupture does not usually cut off blood flow to the heart muscle, at least not directly. Rather, platelets stick to the newly-exposed proteins and clog the artery. The proteins had been hidden inside the plaque, but once exposed to the bloodstream, they prove "foreign" to the platelets, causing activation.

More and more platelets stick — at some point mostly sticking to each other — and the platelets cause activation of other clotting factors in the blood, leading to complete blockage of the artery with a blood clot. A blood clot within a blood vessel is called a **thrombus**.

Normal Artery

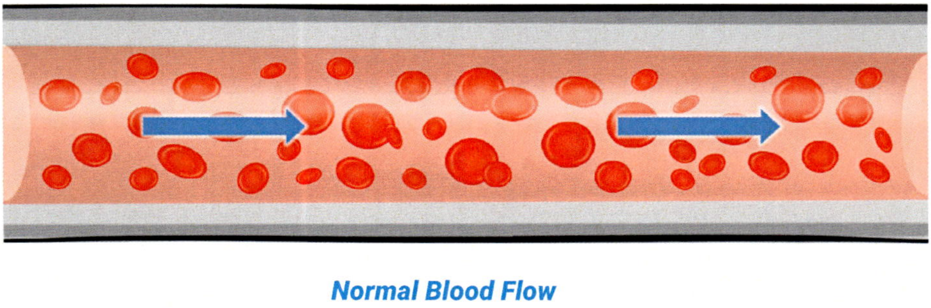

Plaque

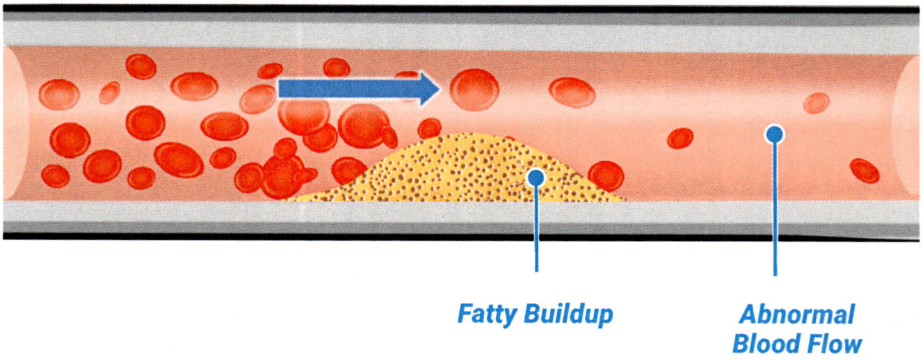

Ruptured Plaque with Thrombus

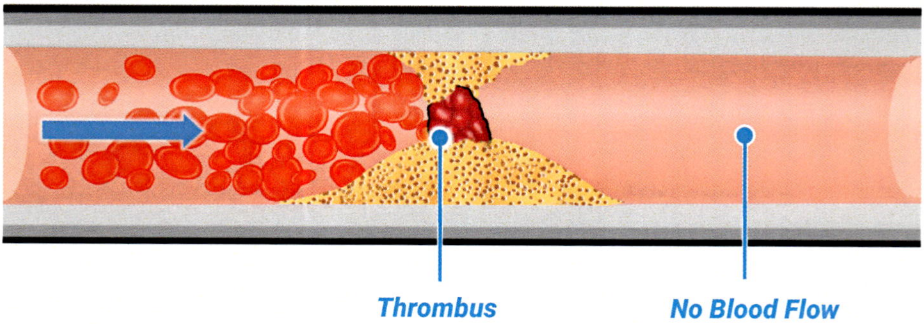

This cascade is why it is important to take **aspirin** if you think you might be having a heart attack, since it could be a STEMI. Aspirin has an anti-platelet effect which helps reduce the activation of the platelets so the platelets do not stick as easily. This effect may help reduce the severity of the blockage and help reduce the damage done by the heart attack.

DO YOU KNOW?

Who invented Aspirin?
No one!

A natural precursor form of aspirin has been used for >3500 years as an herbal remedy. Found in willow bark, it has proven effective for both fever and pain.

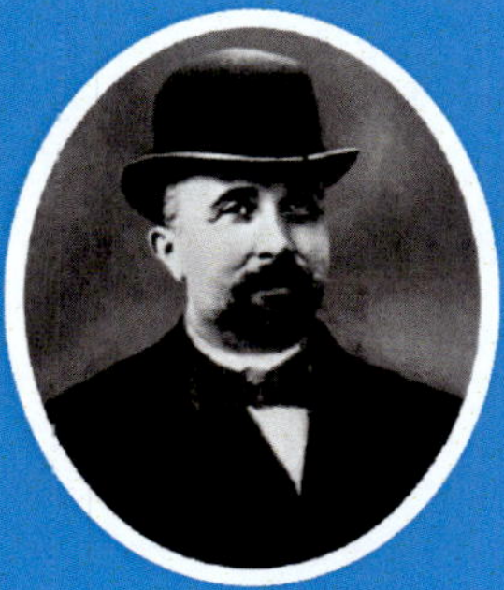

COULD YOU DO THAT?

Acetylsalicylic acid was **synthesized in 1897** by **Felix Hoffmann**, a German chemist at Bayer. It was later named **Aspirin** and marketed as a painkiller, available only by prescription.

Interestingly, 11 days later Hoffmann synthesized a compound known as diamorphone. The substance was found to be an effective cough suppressant; in fact, it was so valuable and *heroic* as a medical aid, Bayer marketed it as an over-the-counter medication they called **Heroin** [32]!

Heroin is now known to be one of the most addictive and dangerous drugs ever discovered, illegal in almost all places, while Aspirin is one of the most widely used medications on earth, available over-the-counter.

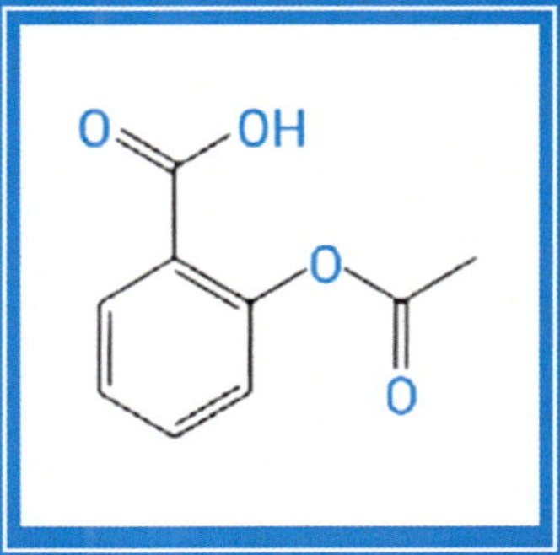

Aspirin chemical structure

It seems there is no shortage of irony when we think of the past through the lens of the present. But my question is: What go-to medications are we using every day *now* which will be banned in the future because they are found to be so detrimental?!

The abrupt blockage of a STEMI is particularly dangerous because often the offending plaque was not severely tight — an artery may only be 60% or 70% blocked prior to plaque rupture. This means the patient may not have experienced symptoms before and may delay seeking care or suffer a delay in diagnosis. Roughly 50% of patients do not know they have blockages of the coronary arteries until they have a heart attack.

A STEMI is also dangerous because a blockage of 60% or 70% will not usually stimulate the development of **collateral arteries**.

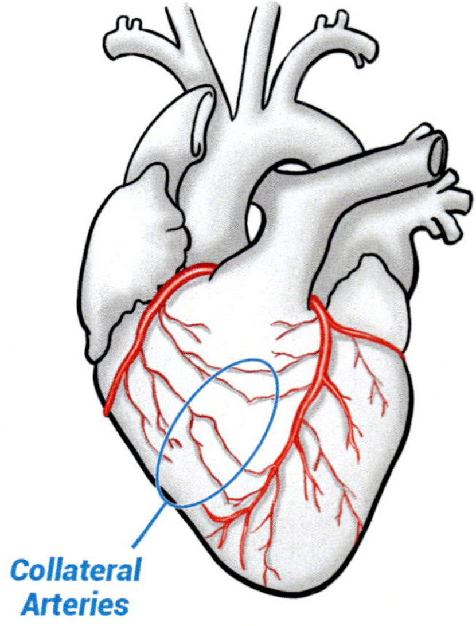

Collateral arteries are tiny connections between the major coronary arteries; they are like single-lane backroads which connect the highways of the major arteries. Under normal conditions, collaterals are present but do not have a role in the delivery of blood to heart muscle.

As a coronary artery becomes blocked, collaterals can "open" and allow some blood flow to the muscle, preventing the myocardial cells from dying. Collaterals take time to develop, probably many days to weeks.

Occasionally a patient tells me a doctor said they have "grown" new arteries after a heart attack. I suppose this isn't completely wrong, but I wonder if patients think they have grown a brand-new, big artery that carries blood in a normal way. This is definitely not the case.

The blood flow through the collateral arteries is not the same as through a major coronary artery; that is, there is much less flow through collaterals than a major coronary artery. The collateral blood flow is often enough to keep the myocardial cells alive, but the flow is not enough when the heart needs to contract more vigorously, such as during **exertion**, which is physical activity.

One study showed the flow through collaterals is only about $1/5$ normal [33]. It's not too surprising the flow is much less: just think of how long it takes for traffic to crawl down a single-lane road when diverted off a big highway!

Collaterals cannot develop fast enough to help during a STEMI.

Without collaterals, the blocked coronary artery is the only route for blood to flow to that area of myocardium, so no blood can get to the muscle. Muscle damage results, which may be extensive and/or severe, leading to weak heart function or even death. Deaths due to STEMI often occur because of **ventricular fibrillation (VF)**.

VF is a "bag of worms" *uncoordinated* contraction of myocardium which does not move blood effectively. It can occur when areas of myocardium are damaged from lack of oxygen, becoming irritable. These areas interfere with the normal transmission of electrical signals.

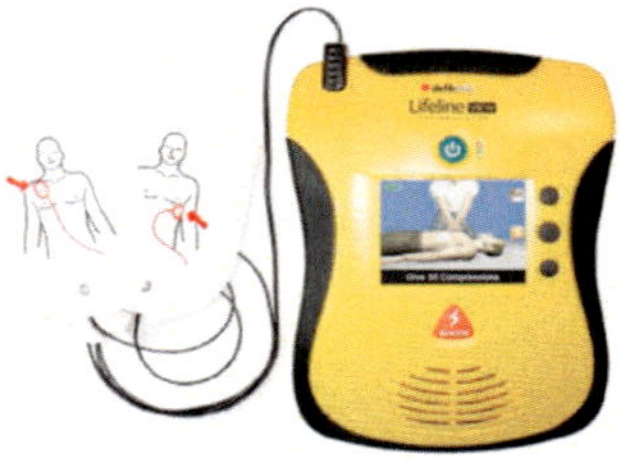

AED

Defibrillation is needed to reset the electrical impulses and thus reset the myocardial contraction. An **AED** is an **A**utomated **E**xternal **D**efibrillator, designed to analyze a person's heart rhythm and deliver an electric shock if VF is detected. Placed at many public venues, AEDs are designed to be used by anyone, without any training. Place the pads on the patient's skin — the pads show you where — and the machine will do the rest.

If you ever think someone is having a heart attack, call 9-1-1 and find an AED. You just might save their life.

TAKE HOME POINTS

Never hesitate to call 9-1-1

& never hesitate to use an AED.

You don't need training for either one!

Generally with STEMI, the longer the artery is blocked, the worse the muscle damage. If the blockage can be relieved very quickly, say, within 30 minutes, there may not be any permanent damage; however, much longer and the damage will likely be irreversible.

Because timely relief of the blockage is crucial, **EMS** (Emergency Medical Services) and hospital programs are trained to identify patients with possible STEMI and get them to a cardiac catheterization lab as soon as possible. The time it takes to get a patient from walking through the door of the ER to when the artery is opened in the cath lab is called the **door-to-balloon time**.

In some cases of STEMI, the disruption of cardiac function is so severe that the entire body is affected. **Cardiogenic shock** occurs when the heart is unable to pump enough blood for other body organs to function properly. With cardiogenic shock, blood pressure is so low that the kidneys, brain, and other organs do not get enough blood flow, and kidney failure or a stroke or other complications can occur. Opening the coronary blockage ASAP is crucial.

Unfortunately, patients with cardiogenic shock can get worse even after the blockage is opened, because the heart is weak and can still struggle to function properly for a while.

A support device such as the **Impella** is used to treat cardiogenic shock; it pumps the blood out of the heart, and while the heart still beats, the heart has less work to do and can relax somewhat and recover. The Impella is placed through the groin or near the collarbone, advanced into the heart and stays in place until the heart is stronger. It can be removed several days later, usually simply by pulling it out in the ICU.

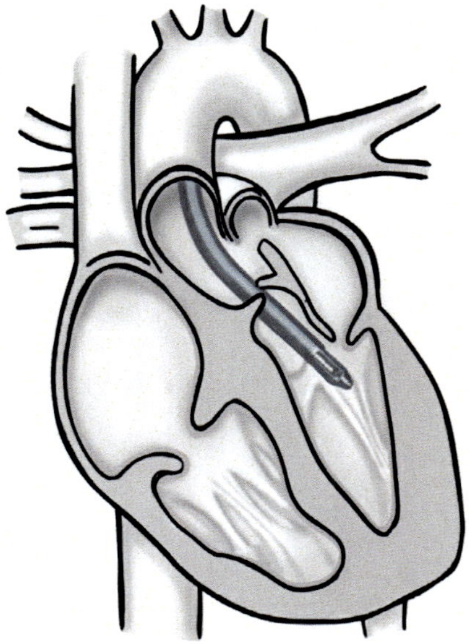

Artist's rendering of Impella inside heart [34]

Prior to the Impella, an **Intra-Aortic Balloon Pump (IABP)** was often used in cases of cardiogenic shock. A "balloon pump" is not quite as effective in treating cardiogenic shock because it does not directly move the blood very much, but it can reduce the amount of work the heart is required to perform and helps improve blood flow through the coronary arteries. Balloon pumps are not used as much anymore in many hospitals, though they continue to be helpful for certain patients.

TAKE HOME POINTS

A STEMI involves sudden & complete blockage of a major coronary artery, leading to myocardial damage due to inadequate collaterals.

A STEMI requires EMERGENT medical care.

A STEMI may be complicated by ventricular fibrillation and cardiogenic shock.

In some cases of STEMI, such as in remote areas or small towns, it may not be feasible to get a patient to a catheterization lab quickly. In such cases, **thrombolytics** may be used to dissolve the thrombus within the artery.

Tissue plasminogen activator, aka **tPA**, is an example of a thrombolytic agent. Given IV, it will act to break down any thrombus in the circulation. Because of its powerful effectiveness in dissolving *any* blood clots, tPA cannot be given to a patient with recent bleeding, surgery or trauma.

NSTEMI

The other major type of heart attack is an **NSTEMI**, which stands for **N**on-**ST** **E**levation **M**yocardial **I**nfarction. It is pronounced "N-STEM-ee." An NSTEMI does not cause a change to the EKG involving the ST segments and often the EKG looks normal.

Unlike STEMI, an NSTEMI does not typically involve rupture of a plaque with activation of platelets, nor does it occur in an artery with a 60% to 70% blockage; rather, it classically involves the worsening of an already-severe blockage, such as a 99% blockage.

An NSTEMI often involves the complete blockage of a small coronary artery or the partial blockage of a major coronary artery. Collaterals may have developed in cases of NSTEMI, such that myocardial damage is often less than in cases of STEMI.

An NSTEMI is not diagnosed from an EKG; rather, it is diagnosed from a rise in cardiac enzymes. **Cardiac enzymes** are chemicals which only occur in heart muscle cells and do not normally circulate in the blood. If the enzymes are detected in the blood, we know that myocardial cells were injured. **Troponin** is one such enzyme commonly checked in suspected cases of NSTEMI.

Treating an NSTEMI is important, but there is not usually a need to open the blockage emergently as with a STEMI, especially if the patient's symptoms have gone away.

TAKE HOME POINTS

An NSTEMI is diagnosed by elevation of cardiac enzymes & requires URGENT medical care.

MORE FLOW, LESS FLOW

Why do heart attacks and heart-attack symptoms often seem to come out of nowhere? No one has a complete answer for the complexity of this disease, but keep in mind that arteries are dynamic— they change from moment to moment — expanding and contracting. Arteries are elastic.

The wall of an artery has 3 main layers.

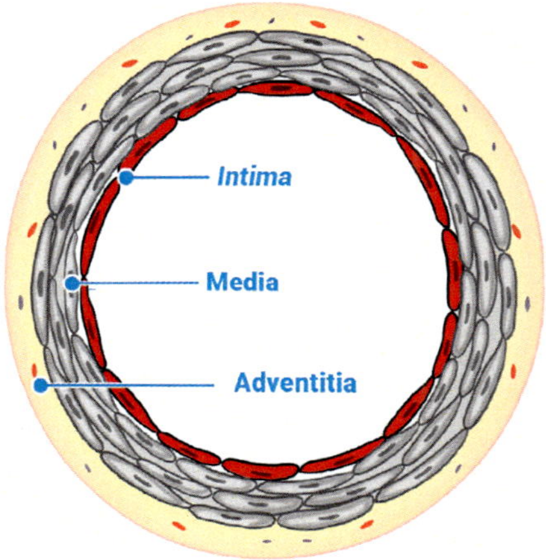

The innermost layer is called the **intima**, which is lined with **endothelial cells** in direct contact with the blood.

The **media** is the middle layer, composed of muscle cells. The muscle in arteries is called **smooth muscle** (in contrast to heart muscle, which is myocardium). The elasticity of the artery wall is due in large part to the smooth muscle within the media.

The outer layer is called the **adventitia**.

DO YOU KNOW?

Which layer of an artery is the strongest: intima, media or adventitia?
Adventitia.

In arteries, the media layer is thickest, while the adventitial layer is strongest. The intima is the thinnest and weakest.

This adventitial strength explains why a plaque may rupture into the lumen (middle) of an artery but not out through the outer wall of the artery. The adventitia is too strong to allow the plaque to burst out of the artery [35].

Arteries tend to expand slightly when the pressure rises and shrink slightly when the pressure lowers. This cycle of expansion and contraction can be felt in the arteries near your wrist or neck and is called your **pulse**.

FOR OVERACHIEVERS & WANNABE PHYSICISTS...

This pulsatile expansion and contraction occurs for the coronary arteries as well. At the risk of losing all but the nerdiest readers, I would like to mention that blood flow (Q) is described by Poiseuille's Law [36]:

Q	Flow rate
P	Pressure
r	Radius
η	Fluid viscosity
l	Length of tubing

$$Q = \frac{\pi P r^4}{8\eta l}$$

Ok, ok — that's the only math equation in the whole book. It is important because it helps show how the elasticity of the arteries is crucial in the body. Follow me for a minute.

Poiseuille's Law basically boils down to this: the factors which control blood flow in an artery are pressure (technically the difference in pressure), viscosity, vessel length, and radius. Stay with me here!

Viscosity is the tendency of "ease" of flow of a liquid. Honey has a high viscosity and water has a relatively low viscosity, for example. Blood has a viscosity slightly higher than water (it's slightly thicker) and its viscosity does not change very much, certainly not in a short period of time. So as far as Poiseuille is concerned, viscosity does not affect blood flow much at all.

The length of blood vessels does not change in a short amount of time.

But the radius of a blood vessel can change in a short time, because arteries are dynamic and elastic. Arteries expand and contract.

And pressure can change.

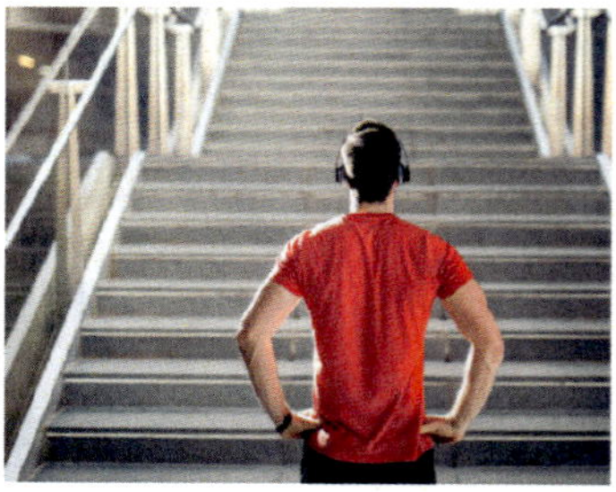

When you decide to walk or run, the skeletal muscles in your legs need more blood. Your heart rate increases, as does the strength of contraction of the myocardium (adrenaline is having an effect on Beta receptors, as you well know!). The myocardium itself needs more oxygen and thus more blood flow in order to keep contracting vigorously. The heart does not have too many options to increase its own blood flow. As you know, it already extracts a high percentage of oxygen from the blood even at rest — typically 75%. The heart cannot lower the viscosity of the blood, and it cannot lengthen the arteries.

But the heart can raise the pressure, which will increase flow. And it can cause the coronary arteries to expand, which will increase flow. To do this, the myocardium releases chemical signals which relax the smooth muscle within the arteries' walls, increasing the size of each

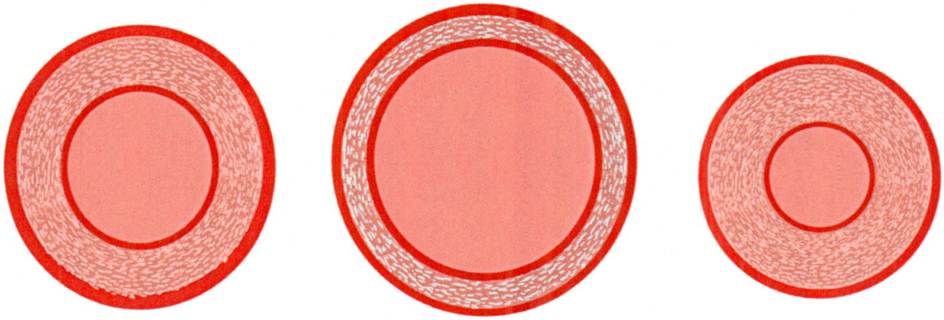

Normal Artery *Vasodilated Artery* *Vasoconstricted Artery*

artery. This increase in size is called **vasodilation**.

This is where Poiseuille's Law becomes important: Blood flow goes up when the size of the artery (the radius) goes up. But blood flow is not proportional to the radius or the radius squared. It's not proportional to the radius to the third power. It is proportional to the radius to the FOURTH power!

I realize this may not be intuitive to a lot of readers, but mathematically, the RADIUS of the artery has a HUGE effect on the blood flow.

In contrast, blood flow is proportional to the pressure to the first power, so an increase in PRESSURE has only a SMALL effect on the blood flow.

As an example, with all other factors stable, if an artery doubles in size, then the blood flow will increase by 16 times! That is incredible to me. Likewise, if an artery increases in size by just 10%, the flow increases by almost 50%. Thus, even small changes in the size of an artery can dramatically affect the blood flow.

$2^{\text{1st power}} = 2$

$2^{\text{2nd power}} = 2 * 2 = 4$

$2^{\text{3rd power}} = 2 * 2 * 2 = 8$

$2^{\text{4th power}} = 2 * 2 * 2 * 2 = 16$

By contrast, small changes in pressure only lead to small changes in flow. If the pressure doubles, the blood flow doubles. If pressure goes up by 10%, the blood flow goes up by 10%.

EXTRA CREDIT $$$

Imagine if you had two bank accounts and you put $100 in each account. One month later, in the account you nicknamed *Pressure* your money has increased by 100 to the first power, so you have $100 more. But in your account *radius*, you have 100 to the fourth power (meaning 100 times 100 times 100 times 100).

How much is that?

$100,000,000! Um, wow. Can I get a radius account at Poiseuille Bank, please?!

This gives an idea how powerful the effect radius has on blood flow — it seems hard to believe because we don't encounter many things in everyday life which correlate to the 4th power.

Consider how hardening of the arteries may play into this process. Let's say your arteries become hardened with calcium and lose their elasticity; as a result, they can't expand or contract much at all.

Now your heart has even fewer options to increase blood flow when needed, because the radius of the arteries cannot change. As usual, viscosity and length of arteries won't change. Pressure can increase, but its effect on blood flow is only modest. So, blood flow to the heart muscle cannot increase very much, no matter how hard the myocardium is forced to work.

This can lead to relatively inadequate blood flow to the heart muscle during exercise, such that you cannot exercise very long without stopping to rest. And that is just because of hardened arteries, not to mention blockages inside the arteries!

The flip side of Poiseuille's Law is also important, that even a small *reduction* in the size of an artery can dramatically *reduce* blood flow. When the smooth muscle in an artery wall contracts and the size of the artery decreases, this change is called **vasoconstriction**. A sudden and persistent vasoconstriction is called **vasospasm**.

Imagine a blockage of 95% inside one of your coronary arteries. The artery is nearly completely blocked, but a trickle of blood still gets through. At rest, enough blood sneaks past the blockage to keep your heart muscle functioning and free from damage.

But then you go outside into the cold on a winter evening. As an automatic response to avoid losing heat, the arteries in your skin constrict and decrease in size (this constriction is due to your old friend the sympathetic nervous system — and, yes, your body reacts to freezing cold the same as fighting a snake/lawyer).

The arteries of your heart also constrict and get smaller. As you now know, even a small decrease in the size can reduce the blood flow a lot. The vasoconstriction may cause the 95% blockage to become 100%, completely cutting off blood flow to the muscle.

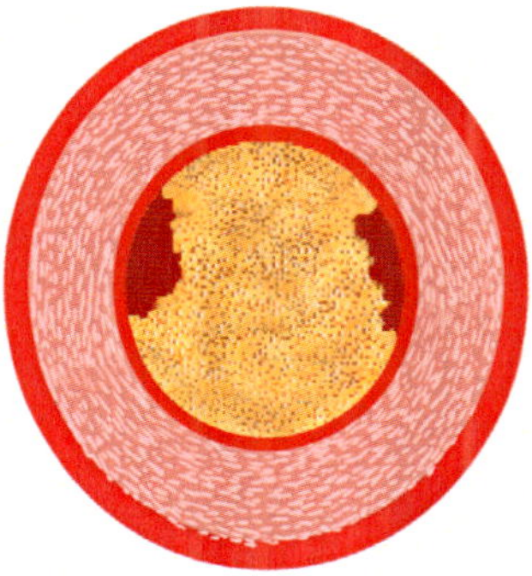

Artery with 95% Plaque

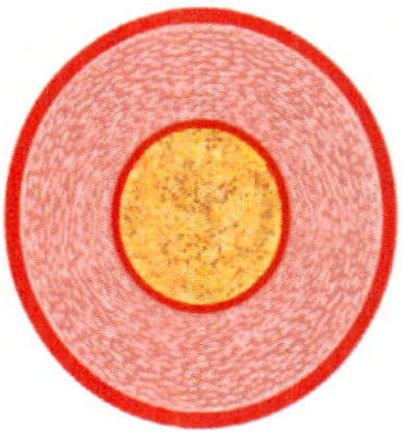

Vasoconstricted Artery with occlusion

With a complete blockage, the myocardium has no oxygen to use — yet it must keep beating for you to stay alive — so **anaerobic metabolism** kicks in and lactic acid and other metabolic by-products build up; this results in pain or discomfort.

A heart attack may result if the complete blockage is not relieved, since anaerobic metabolism cannot be used for very long by myocardial cells.

The fix for the complete blockage in this situation is simply for the artery to relax again, since the blockage itself did not truly change, just the size of the artery and the available space for blood to flow past the blockage.

Thus, it is advantageous to keep coronary arteries as relaxed and vasodilated as possible whenever CAD is present.

TAKE HOME POINTS

Blood flow is proportional to artery radius to the 4th power & pressure to the 1st power.

Thus, changes in artery SIZE have a HUGE effect on blood flow while PRESSURE changes have only a SMALL effect.

Hardening of arteries can impair blood flow by impairing vasodilation.

JUST RELAX!

How can you relax an artery?

Nitroglycerin. The body converts nitroglycerin to nitric oxide, which relaxes smooth muscle, causing the arterial walls to expand and arteries to increase in size. This increase in size helps more blood flow through the arteries.

Chest pain due to coronary artery disease improves with nitroglycerin because more oxygen is delivered to the muscle, reducing anaerobic metabolism and decreasing the production of lactic acid.

Nitroglycerin is not a pain-killer (analgesic) per se and does not interfere with pain signals but rather helps relieve the process causing the pain. As you now know, even a small increase in the size of the artery can allow a dramatic increase in the blood flow (thank you, Poiseuille). And when blood flow is impaired, even a little improvement helps.

When a patient has chest pain, he or she will often be advised to take nitroglycerin in a form which dissolves under the tongue. This under-the-tongue, or sublingual, method gets the nitroglycerin into the bloodstream and working faster than swallowing the pill and waiting until it is absorbed in the stomach.

Strangely, nitroglycerin is also used as a component of many types of explosives. Alfred Nobel used nitroglycerin in his invention dynamite in 1867. He was later prescribed nitroglycerin for chest pain in 1896, shortly before his death. How unusual — for a substance to have both healing and destructive power.

Of note, nitroglycerin in solid form is quite stable and will NOT explode under your tongue or inside your chest!

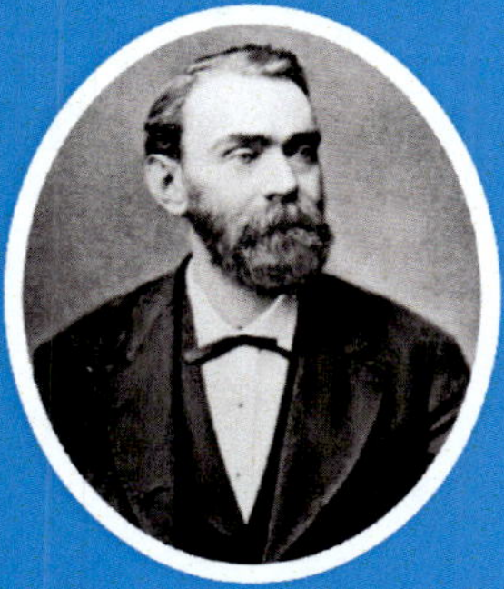

COULD YOU DO THAT?

Alfred Nobel was a Swedish chemist and businessman who held 355 patents. He read his own obituary which described him as the "**merchant of death**," mistakenly written after his brother died. The moniker distressed him so much that he established the **Nobel Prize**, hoping to be remembered as a champion of life and humanity and not remembered for his destructive ingenuity [37].

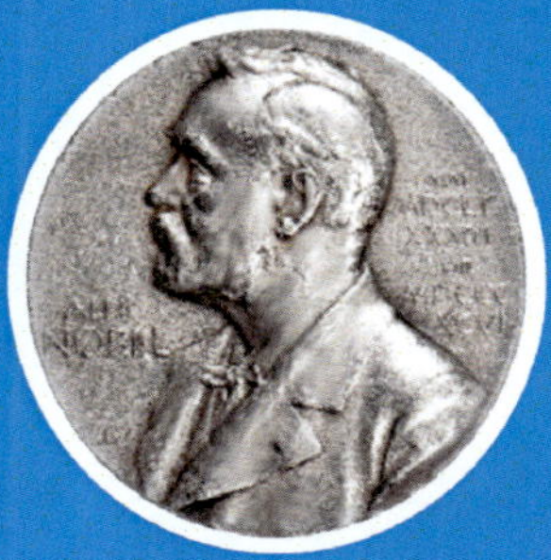

Just as cold conditions can cause coronary vasospasm and thus a reduction in coronary blood flow, exercise and intense emotional distress can do the same thing. So, be careful when exercising on a cold day while upset! You may want to take the precaution of bringing some dynamite with you to put under your tongue. Well, ok, it might be best to just stick with nitroglycerin.

Interestingly, it is possible for emotions alone to cause coronary vasospasm, resulting in angina or even a myocardial infarction [38]. It seems even though you can't consciously control your heart, you can subconsciously affect it!

SYMPTOMS

Does chest pain always mean someone is having a heart attack? Nah. But chest pain could be an indicator of coronary artery disease (CAD), and it is important to pay attention to any symptoms you may have.

The classic symptom associated with CAD is called **angina pectoris**. Most people shorten this to angina. The term comes from a Latin root word that means "strangling." It was originally described by Dr. William Heberden in 1768 as a "sense of strangling and anxiety," [39] though he did not link the symptom specifically to heart disease. His successor Dr. Edward Jenner made the connection of angina with narrowing of the coronary arteries [40].

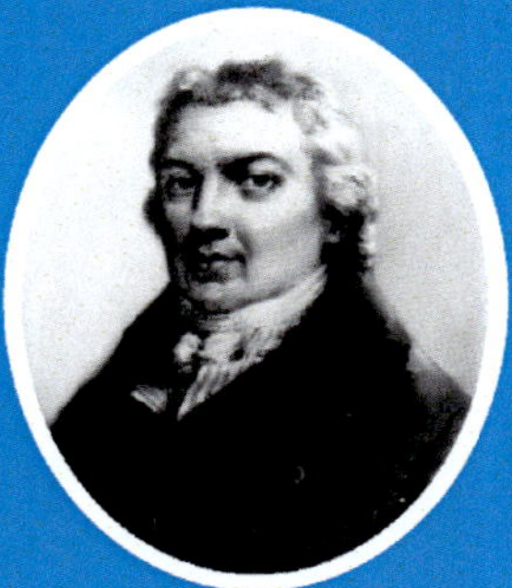

COULD YOU DO THAT?

Dr. Edward Jenner, British physician and surgeon, in addition to making keen observations and insights on the heart, developed the world's **first vaccine**. He used **cowpox** to inoculate an **eight-year-old boy** against smallpox. The word "vaccine" comes from Latin *vaccinus* which means "from cows." Due to pioneering the concept of vaccination, Dr. Jenner is said to have **saved more human lives than any person in history** [41].

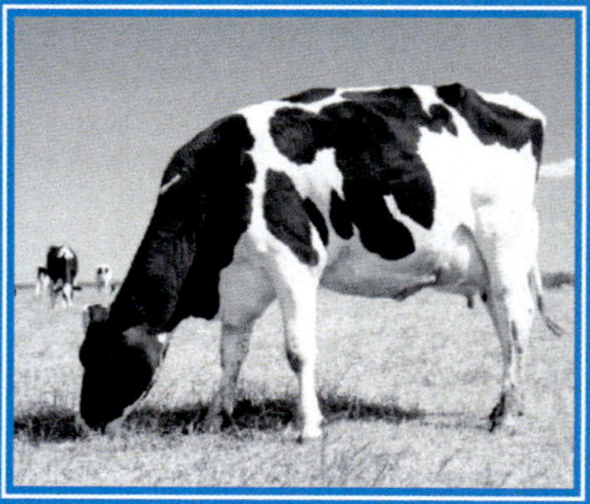

Angina is often described by patients as a "pressure" or heaviness of the chest — as "an elephant sitting on my chest." When I ask patients about their symptoms, it is common for them to insist that they never had "pain" but instead had discomfort or pressure or heaviness.

Remember the sympathetic nerve fibers and the vagus nerve? The sympathetic fibers arise from ganglia, which are like tiny nerve centers that exist outside the brain. These fibers interact with the nerves of the ribs of the upper chest.

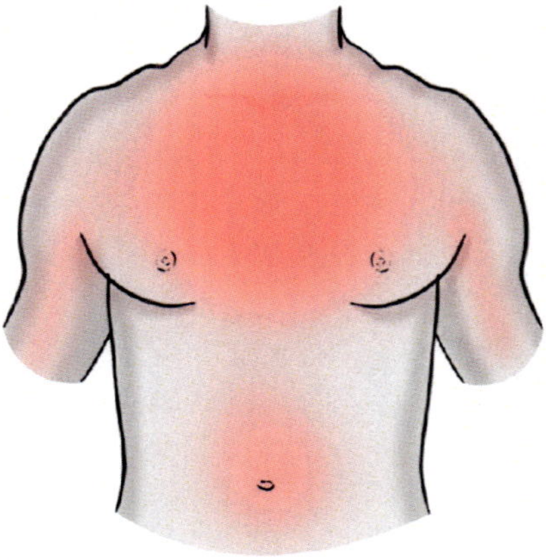

Affected areas

The point is that when these nerves become activated, the pain signal extends across the whole band of tissue, the whole length of any affected rib. This seems to be why patients often experience a "band" of discomfort across the chest and not only on the left side, where the heart is located.

This wide-spread distribution of discomfort is fairly consistent and can be helpful in the evaluation of patients. When patients point with one finger to the site of their chest pain, they are not very likely to be having a heart attack [42]. By contrast, when patients hold a clenched fist over their chest, called **Levine's sign**, they have around an 80% chance of having ischemia [43].

The activation of sympathetic fibers often causes patients to experience nausea and excessive sweating (the medical term is **diaphoresis**) along with angina.

Pain or discomfort from the heart often extends to other areas of the body. Often the left arm or shoulder may be involved, because they are also served by the sympathetic fibers near the top of the chest. An important point is that the arm is not in any danger, and the blood flow to the arm is fine — it is only cross-talk between the nerve fibers that misleads the brain into thinking pain is coming from the shoulder or arm.

Patients often experience anginal discomfort that seems similar to heart-burn, perhaps more of a burning discomfort than a pressure; in fact, some patients misinterpret angina as heart-burn.

Remember how the vagus nerve "wanders" through the chest, serving many organs including the GI tract? Given this information, it is not surprising that angina can be mistaken for heart-burn because the nerve fibers are shared between the heart and the stomach.

For some patients, heart-related pain may also extend into the neck or jaw or back or to the right arm.

In addition to angina, patients may experience shortness of breath. Some patients will term this "catching my breath" or feeling "winded." The shortness of breath may occur instead of angina or along with it.

Some patients experience no symptoms. Some studies indicate up to 75% of people with CAD do not experience angina [44].

Patients with diabetes can be among those with barely noticeable or mild symptoms. Some diabetic patients have *no* symptoms; in fact, around 25% of heart attacks are "silent" or cause no symptoms in diabetic patients [44]. Neuropathy is a common complication of diabetes, where nerves do not transmit signals normally and patients have dull sensation or no sensation at all. This neuropathy classically affects the feet and lower extremities but it can affect the nerves of the chest. Neuropathy may be part of why diabetic patients often do not have much chest discomfort with CAD.

Women may have classic symptoms but also experience less recognizable symptoms such as anxiety, a sense of unease, or fatigue.

SYMPTOMS of Coronary Artery Disease

Chest Pain	**Shortness of breath**
Chest Pressure	**Windedness**
Neck Pain	**Heartburn**
Jaw Pain	**Nausea**
Arm Pain	**Anxiety**
Shoulder Pain	

No symptoms at all

There is little connection between the severity of heart damage and the pain experienced by the patient [45]. Small blockages can cause severe pain and extensive damage can sometimes be asymptomatic.

Anginal symptoms characteristically occur with exertion and resolve with rest. This means that a person may have no symptoms while resting but begin having discomfort when walking or going up stairs. After stopping to rest, the symptoms go away. Such a pattern is textbook for angina. In addition to rest, nitroglycerin can often speed up the resolution of angina.

Angina which follows this textbook pattern is called **stable angina**. If angina symptoms occur at rest or become very frequent — more than the patient previously experienced — or if pain does not resolve with nitroglycerin, the symptoms are called **unstable angina**. Unstable angina is even more concerning than stable angina and may signal severe CAD or an impending heart attack. Pain due to a heart attack usually does NOT go away with rest or with nitroglycerin [46].

Be sure to let your physician know if you have changes in symptoms or any new symptoms. And if you have chest pain which does not resolve with rest or nitroglycerin, seek medical attention immediately.

TAKE HOME POINTS

Severe chest pain is concerning.

Nah, not exactly... Any chest symptom is concerning!

Be careful not to dismiss what you feel.

Tell your doctor about *anything* abnormal you are experiencing.

HOW DID THIS HAPPEN?

The build-up of plaque in the arteries is thought to take many years, in changing from a normal artery to a severe blockage.

The general term for thickening and hardening of the arteries is **arteriosclerosis**. This is usually due to the build-up of plaque. Arteries lose their elasticity and become stiff.

Almost any artery is susceptible to this process of plaque build-up, but commonly affected arteries are:

ARTERY LOCATION	DISEASE	COMPLICATION
Heart	**Coronary Artery Disease**	**Heart Attack**
Neck	**Carotid Artery Disease**	**Stroke**
Kidneys	**Renal Artery Stenosis**	**High Blood Pressure**
Legs	**Peripheral Artery Disease**	**Pain with Walking**

Interestingly, this process does not occur in the veins of the body [46]. There is no such thing as Coronary Vein Disease. Veins have problems and diseases, but they do not get clogged with plaque. However, if veins are used as conduit for bypass surgery, they develop plaque! It is likely the **wall stress** involved in carrying blood at high pressures affects the vein repair process, leading to the build-up of plaque and "veinosclerosis."

One of the first signs of arteriosclerosis is the **fatty streak**, an area of whitish discoloration on the inside of an artery. This abnormal collection of cells is likely related to inflammation. Most children in first-world countries older than 10 years have fatty streaks in their arteries, evidence this disease process starts when we are young.

As a person ages, this fatty streak matures and becomes a plaque as more elements are added to it – mostly fats, cholesterol, and calcium.

The plaque buildup can become so thick that it decreases the space available for blood to flow and may completely block an artery. The plaque may become hardened and calcified.

The exact mechanism of how this process happens is not well-understood. However, several factors have been identified which are closely associated with plaque formation.

Damage to the lining of the arteries can set off a process which ultimately leads to plaque accumulation and blockages. All of your blood vessels are lined with special cells called **endothelial cells**, collectively called endothelium. These cells have the tricky role of maintaining blood flow within the arteries while also maintaining the strength and integrity of the arterial wall. To do this, endothelial cells are constantly releasing certain chemicals into the blood and absorbing certain chemicals from the blood. Thank God this finely balanced process doesn't require any mental effort! Your endothelial cells bring order to the chaotic movement of your blood, and, like all the cells in your body, they are unique to you.

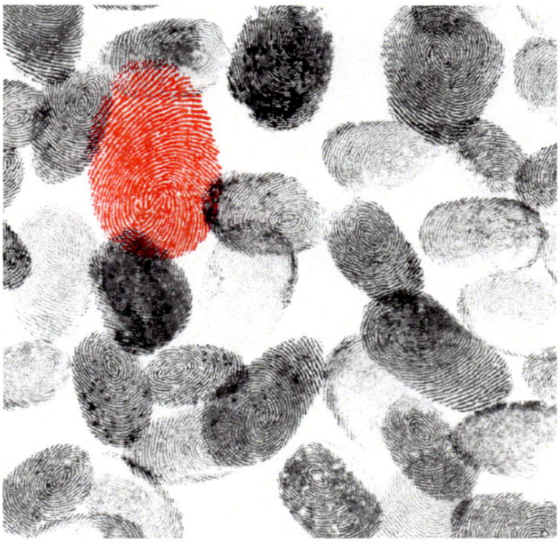

I think of the endothelium a bit like skin: it's got to keep particular things in and specific things out. Any break in the skin must be repaired or many problems will result, including bleeding. Similarly, any break in your blood vessels must be repaired, which is a function of your endothelial cells.

The endothelium releases chemicals which signal an injury has occurred and repair is needed. Cells mobilize within your blood to the area in preparation for repair. But, if during this process there are a lot of fats and cholesterol circulating, these particles can incidentally enter the site of injury, thereby contributing to the build-up of plaque.

Stop and think about your blood for a minute: In all human history, no substitute for blood has ever been found or invented.

Humans went to the moon and you can call Siberia using a computer held in your hand, but blood has proven too complex to engineer. It is so complex that it circulates for years on end and never (fully) stops – because if it does all stop, you die. But some of it will stop and clot if you get a tiny cut. You don't tell your blood when you get cut or where you get cut. Your endothelium and your blood "figure" it out, find the defect, and plug it – all without plugging up the whole artery with blood clots.

If it were not for God's amazing design, you would have bled to death with your first papercut. Or all of your blood would have clotted. Thank God for all the things we never think about!

Causes of damage to your arteries include:

SMOKING

There are more than 7,000 chemicals in cigarette smoke [47]. Over 250 of these chemicals are known to be toxic and include arsenic, a known poison; ethylene oxide, used to make antifreeze; and formaldehyde, used to preserve dead tissues.

Carbon monoxide is also present in cigarette smoke, which is a colorless and odorless by-product of combustion; it binds >200 times more readily to hemoglobin than oxygen does [48]. Carbon monoxide can be deadly when a person is exposed to it in an enclosed space, such as a garage.

These chemicals cause damage to the endothelial cells lining the arteries, contributing to the development of CAD; these chemicals also cause damage to many other tissues in the body.

To reiterate, the chemicals in cigarette smoke do not only impair healing, they actively CAUSE damage.

DO YOU KNOW?

How many cigarettes per day does it take to increase your risk of CAD?
One!

Smoking only ONE cigarette per day can DOUBLE the risk of CAD [49].

If you have ever smoked cigarettes, the best thing you can do for your health is **never smoke again**. There can be positive changes in your body within 24 hours[50].

TAKE HOME POINTS

Stay away from cigarettes.

Your heart & every part of your body will thank you.

HIGH BLOOD PRESSURE AKA HYPERTENSION

High blood pressure can cause arteries to stiffen and lose elasticity. These changes allow plaque to more easily develop. In addition, high blood pressure forces the heart muscle to work harder since your myocardium creates your blood pressure.

When high blood pressure is present over a sustained period of time, the heart muscle cells **hypertrophy**, meaning the cells increase in size (they do not increase in number – remember, myocardial cells cannot be replaced or new ones added!). Thus, the walls of the heart become thicker.

This may not sound so bad, but blood and oxygen cannot move as well through the thick myocardium. New capillaries do not grow when the muscle hypertrophies, so oxygen must diffuse a greater distance from the capillaries to the myocardial cells, sacrificing some of the metabolic efficiency of the heart.

In addition to these troubles for the heart, chronic high blood pressure can cause complications other organs, such as the kidneys, brain and eyes.

DO YOU KNOW?

What animal has the highest blood pressure?
A heart surgeon who is told his/her case is delayed.

The redness of the face correlates with the blood pressure to the 1st power.

Meanwhile, a giraffe's normal blood pressure can reach 300/180 mmHg, the highest among all non-surgeon vertebrates [24].

If you have high blood pressure, it is important to work with your Primary Care Physician or Cardiologist to develop and follow a plan to maintain your blood pressure in a healthy range.

DIABETES

Chronically high levels of sugar in your blood can cause endothelial cells to malfunction; the endothelial cells have difficulty sending the proper chemical signals in correct amounts. This dysfunction allows damage to the intima of the coronary arteries and interferes with proper healing, contributing to the build-up of plaque.

Diabetes can be due to the pancreas not producing enough insulin, known as **Type 1**. Diabetes can also be due to insulin resistance, where cells in the body do not respond to insulin normally, resulting in **Type 2**.

DO YOU KNOW?

How much does Type I diabetes increase the risk of dying from CAD, compared to patients without diabetes? 11 Times.

Type II diabetes increases the risk 3 times [51].

Other factors associated with atherosclerosis do not cause damage directly to your endothelium but can interfere with the endothelial repair process. These include:

HIGH CHOLESTEROL

Cholesterol is necessary for life, as a component of cell membranes and as a building block for other molecules, such as steroids.

Cholesterol is a complex molecule which disintegrates when exposed to blood, so it travels inside another molecule. The molecule which transports cholesterol to the body's cells is called **Low-Density Lipoprotein** aka **LDL**.

LDL is called "bad cholesterol" because high levels of LDL can be associated with severe build-up of plaque.

EXTRA CREDIT

LDL is not cholesterol; it is a lipoprotein. So it is technically incorrect to call LDL "bad cholesterol," though almost everyone does.

I think of LDL as being like an overloaded cholesterol trash-bag, prone to dropping and spilling cholesterol at any moment, at any cell nearby. If there is an injury in the artery wall, LDL may drop cholesterol there, contributing to plaque formation.

High-Density Lipoprotein, or **HDL**, carries cholesterol away from the body's cells; it takes cholesterol to the liver, where the cholesterol is directed into bile. Bile goes into the small intestine to help dissolve food.

HDL is called "good cholesterol" because high levels of HDL may be associated with reduced build-up of plaque (though like LDL, HDL is a lipoprotein).

I think of HDL like a cholesterol vacuum cleaner, ready to suck up cholesterol and take it to the liver for disposal.

In general, it is desirable to have low LDL levels and high HDL levels.

TAKE HOME POINTS

You want to have low LDL [52]
& high HDL.

Every animal cell has the ability to make cholesterol, so humans do not need to get any cholesterol from food. We get no cholesterol from plants we eat, but we do absorb cholesterol from animal products.

The medical term for high cholesterol is **hypercholesterolemia**. For many years, it was assumed a diet high in meat, eggs, and dairy products, caused hypercholesterolemia. This assumption has been questioned in recent years[53], and while the regulation of cholesterol in the body is complicated, recent studies show that consuming cholesterol does not raise levels in the blood very much for most people [54]. Interestingly, vegetarians can have high cholesterol levels.

There is a genetic component to the metabolism of cholesterol. Familial hypercholesterolemia, which affects 1 in 250 Americans, can cause such high levels that cholesterol collects in yellowish areas around the eyes and knees, elbows, and knuckles [55].

Often cholesterol can be managed with lifestyle modifications, while **statin medications** are used if medical therapy is needed.

HIGH TRIGLYCERIDES

Triglycerides are complex molecules which the body uses to store energy as fat. If you eat food and your body does not use the calories at that time, your body converts the fatty molecules in the food to triglycerides, which are transported to fat stores. This is part of why eating late at night contributes to obesity, because you are not "working off" the calories soon after eating.

High levels of triglycerides have been associated with the build-up of plaque in the coronary arteries, so work with your physician(s) on a plan to manage your triglyceride levels.

FAMILY HISTORY

CAD often "runs" in families. This can be due to behavioral factors such as unhealthy patterns of diet and exercise and can also be due to genetic factors. The actual mechanism of how genetics affects atherosclerosis is an area of active research [56].

TAKE HOME POINTS

Choose your parents carefully!

LACK OF EXERCISE

There is a strong relationship between a lack of exercise and CAD [57], though exactly how lack of exercise contributes to the development of plaque is not clear. A habitual pattern of lack of exercise or physical exertion is known as a **sedentary lifestyle**.

Any physical activity is better than none (barring injury or physical disability), and it is recommended that we all get at least 30 minutes of vigorous exercise 4-5 times per week. Walking from the couch to the kitchen refrigerator does not count!

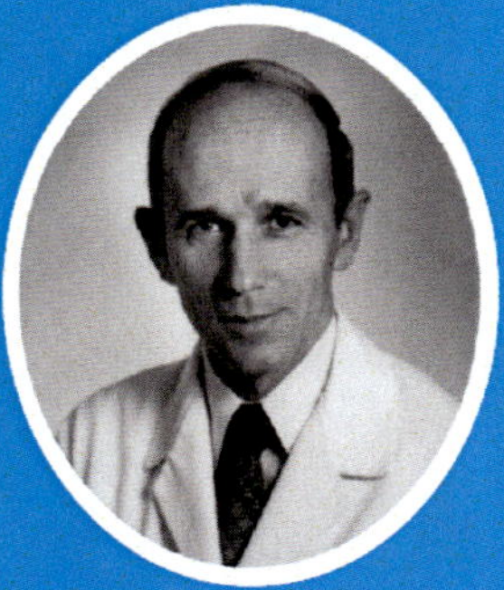

COULD YOU DO THAT?

Dr. Kenneth Cooper coined the term **Aerobics** in the title of his 1968 book, which sold millions of copies. He pioneered preventive medicine at the **Cooper Clinic** in Dallas, TX [58]. He was called before the Board of the Dallas County Medical Society due to the establishment's concerns vigorous physical activity was unsafe and would kill people. He overcame the obstacles and numerous studies later proved people **live longer** with aerobic exercise, just like he said. He has also written about how faith plays an important role in good health [59].

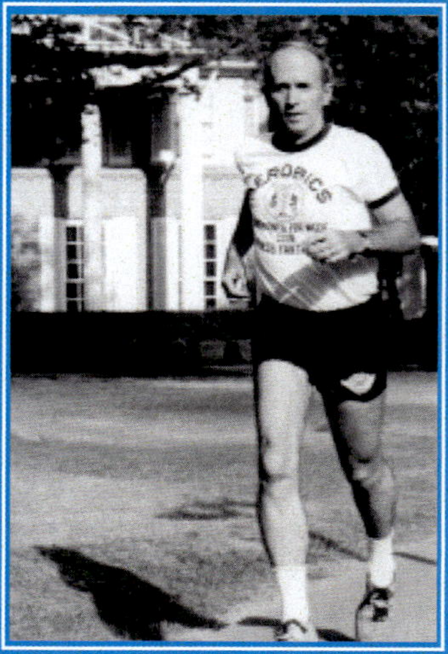

ADVANCED AGE

The risk of CAD increases with age. About 80% of Americans over age 80 can be expected to have some evidence of cardiovascular disease [60].

Meanwhile, reader of advanced age, don't sell yourself short: While the overall life-expectancy from birth for all races in the US is roughly 78 years, the life expectancy of an 80 year-old is 9 years [61]!

This means on average, an 80 year-old will live to be 89 years old. This info seems counter-intuitive but I think of it like the people who reach 80 years have already out-lived peers who died at an earlier age, proving a certain physical and mental fortitude allowing continued well-being.

There are other factors thought to contribute to atherosclerosis but have an unclear relationship with CAD. These factors include:

CHRONIC STRESS

Emotional or physical tension experienced over a prolonged period of time likely contributes to CAD. People who feel stressed on an on-going basis may engage unhealthy behaviors such as smoking, consuming alcohol or overeating. In addition, there are likely poorly-understood aspects of chronic stress which contribute to the development of plaque.

PERSONALITY

Certain personality traits have been associated with an increased risk of CAD, including excessive drive, ambition, and aggressiveness — the so-called Type A personality [44].

Conversely, long-standing optimism has been shown to be associated with *reduced* risk of CAD in the elderly [62].

IMMUNE SYSTEM

The immune system seems to have a role in the regulation of the endothelium and the development of CAD. Patients on immunosuppressants after heart transplantation can develop CAD at an early age, even when the transplanted heart came from a young donor. In addition, people with immune conditions such as Crohn's disease, ulcerative colitis and lupus may be at increased risk of CAD.

The mechanism by which the immune system regulates the coronary arteries is not well-understood and is an area of active research.

SLEEP APNEA

Sleep apnea is a sleep disorder characterized by the brief stoppage of breathing during sleep; it is often marked by snoring and typically affects overweight or obese people. Oxygen levels can decrease during sleep for people with sleep apnea, which may contribute to cellular stress of the endothelium, thereby contributing to atherosclerosis.

Even aside from sleep apnea, simply getting inadequate amounts of sleep has been associated with increased risk of CAD [63].

OBESITY

Obesity is an independent risk factor for CAD. Obesity

is usually defined as a **Body Mass Index** or **BMI** > 30. The BMI is calculated as the person's mass in kg divided by height in meters, squared. There are numerous on-line calculators you can use to check your BMI.

Other measures such as waist circumference can also be helpful in gauging obesity. Over 80% of patients with CAD are overweight or obese [64].

Often patients lose 10-15 lbs of weight over the course of treatment with CABG. Be one who uses the weight loss as a jump-start to establishing a new, healthier body weight!

ALCOHOL INTAKE

It is unclear how alcohol intake affects CAD. A small amount of alcohol intake such as one drink per day has historically not been thought to harm the heart, although recent evidence suggests *any* alcohol intake may be detrimental [65]. More conclusively, *heavy* alcohol intake is *definitely* associated with heart disease, and alcohol has a direct toxic effect on myocardial cells [66].

For most patients, the development of Coronary Artery Disease (CAD) involves a combination of these factors. Still, some patients develop CAD without any obvious risk factors.

LETS GET PERSONAL

What about you?
What risk factors apply to you?

There are surely other factors not yet identified which contribute to atherosclerosis. Could infections lead to CAD? There have been reports of Herpes virus being correlated with the development of CAD [67]. Could living in the South contribute to CAD? Getting a tattoo? Having been born by C-section? Will COVID affect the development of CAD? It will be interesting to see what insights we may learn in the future regarding this complex disease.

Only one risk factor can never be changed — family history. And there is no known way to stop the passage of time, so your age is continuously advancing. But everything else can possibly be affected by your choices. When it comes to striving for good health, it is useful to work on improving these modifiable factors.

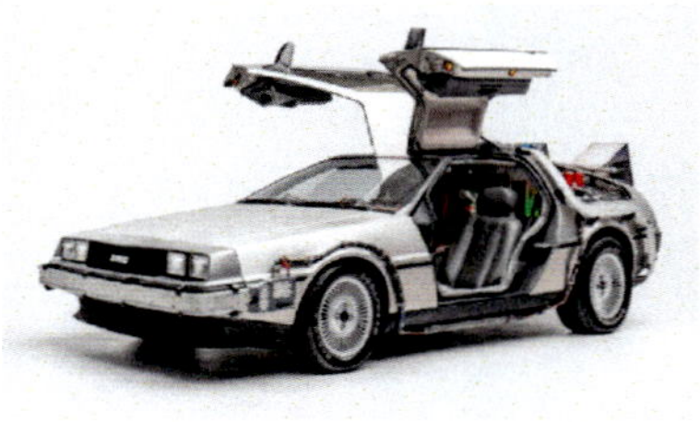

We all know we cannot change the past. Yet when a crisis comes, we often dwell on past mistakes, past failures. What if I had exercised more? What if I had eaten better? These are questions worth pondering, to figure out how to make better choices in the future. But there is no benefit in obsessing about the past.

More effective questions are: What can I do now? How can I change? Instead of blaming yourself or others, consider what positive choices you can make now. Use your mental energy on something you can do now, not wasting mental energy on the past, which cannot be altered.

So, what can you do? What choices can you make? Are you prepared to commit yourself to better health?

TAKE HOME POINTS

YOU are responsible for your own health & YOU can decide to live a healthier life TODAY.

If you are a smoker, the first thing to do is stop smoking. Right now. It is not an easy task. Make the choice and commit to it. As detailed in the excellent book **Atomic Habits**[68], don't say you are trying to quit smoking; instead, say "I am a non-smoker." This small shift in thinking and speaking will help make you successful, allowing you to identify with a desired behavior rather than an undesired one.

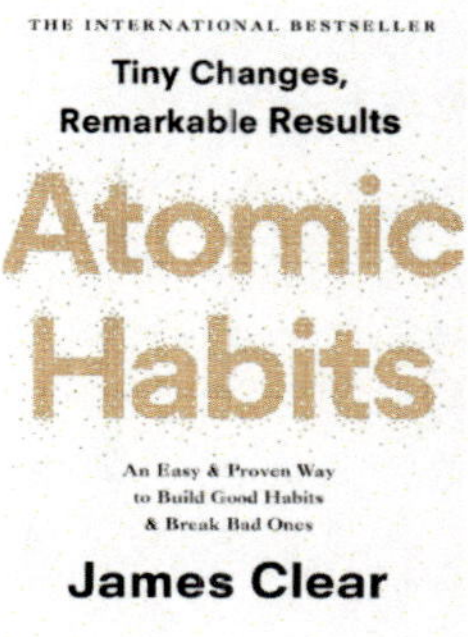

Another technique is to make positive impressions on your subconscious mind, such as when you fall asleep at night [69]. For instance, as you fall asleep, concentrate on phrases such as "I am thankful that I have stopped smoking" or "I am looking forward to waking up tomorrow and breathing better." These kinds of messages can have a positive effect on your mind and body in unexplained ways.

Get help from your doctor to make it happen, if needed. For many people, cigarette smoking is a combination of a habit and an addiction (to nicotine). There are techniques and products which can help with both, such as holding an alternative in your hand like a pen or straw when feeling the urge to smoke, as well as nicotine patches and gum for symptoms of withdrawal. Fortunately, urges and symptoms fade over time for almost all people.

Your family needs to help; they want you to be successful. If your spouse smokes, ask if him or her to stop along with you because otherwise the frequent exposure to the trigger will reduce your chance of success. A patient once told me he quit because he made a deal with his 8 year-old grand-daughter: she promised to never start smoking, if he promised to never smoke again. What a great deal! Never smoking again is the best choice you can make for your health. You and your loved ones — perhaps even your grandchildren — will benefit.

Can you exercise more? Start where you are. If you do not exercise, I suggest committing yourself to taking the stairs down one floor. If you're going up one floor, take the elevator. Going down two floors, take the elevator. But going down one floor? Take the stairs. It is

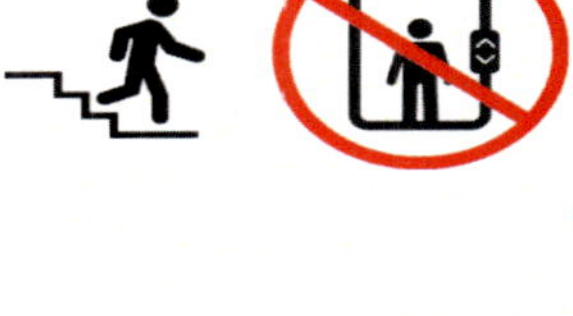

a small bit of exercise and helpful to your body. And you may find yourself taking the stairs to go up a floor before too long. Or taking the stairs down two floors. Your effort can gain momentum and the small change will compound over time to create a noticeable result. Keep in mind that any physical activity is better than none!

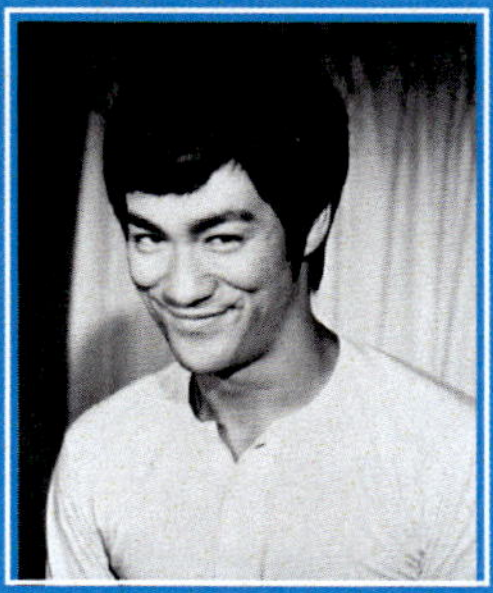

COULD YOU DO THAT?

The kung-fu guru and actor **Bruce Lee** pretty-much **never took the elevator**, according to his daughter Shannon Lee. In the rare instance where an elevator simply could not be avoided, he did **push-ups** while waiting for the elevator! [70]

I have found this to be true in my own life. About a year ago, I decided to take the stairs down one floor. Now, I almost always use the stairs no matter how many flights up or down; some days, I'll go up twelve flights of stairs to get to the top floor of the hospital. Some days I don't! I don't beat myself up about it if I take the elevator. I am satisfied in knowing I am a lot more physically active now than a year ago. It started with a simple change.

I understand some patients can't exercise due to physical limitations such as arthritis or a bad hip or bad back. Certainly, some people cannot go up and down stairs. Or do push-ups. Just do the best with what you've got. Consider water exercises if your joints are an issue. Work out your arms if your hips and knees are bad. Move some part of your body! Work out your eyelids if you have to.

What can you adjust about your diet? I may be a dietician's worst nightmare but my advice on diet is to make small, healthy choices you can keep up the rest of your life. In my opinion, **small, sustainable choices** are better than trying to revolutionize your diet and then failing after a short time, going back to the same old unhealthy habits.

After he underwent bypass surgery, an 80 year-old patient of mine admitted he had eaten 4 slices of bacon every day of his life, since he was a young

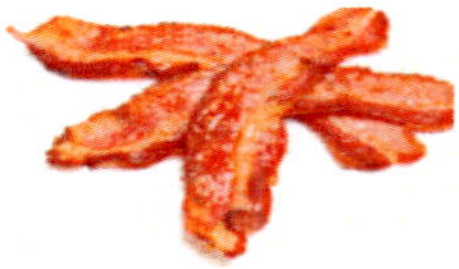

boy. Some dieticians would no doubt tell him he couldn't eat bacon anymore. But not me. My advice was for him to eat 3 slices of bacon every day. It is a small choice, but a healthy one, at least compared to his usual habit. And likely doable for the rest of his life.

Who knows? Over time, he may lose a bit of weight, have a bit more energy, and decide it is worth it to go to 2 slices of bacon a day. And then one. And then perhaps every other day. Small choices compounded over years can have a dramatic effect, whereas revolutionary changes only sustained for a short time have little lasting effect. In fact, many people gain more weight back than they lost after "going on a diet."

Another issue is salt intake. In general, your body does not need much salt and most Americans consume way too much salt. It is helpful and healthy to consume less salt. Most patients do not need to cut out *all* salt, they just need to consume **less salt**. For most patients, I recommend cooking food with as little salt as you can and then **do not add salt at the table**. Caveat: If you have a very weak heart, heart failure, or kidney problems, then you may need to follow a truly no-salt diet. As always, follow the personalized advice and recommendation of your physician.

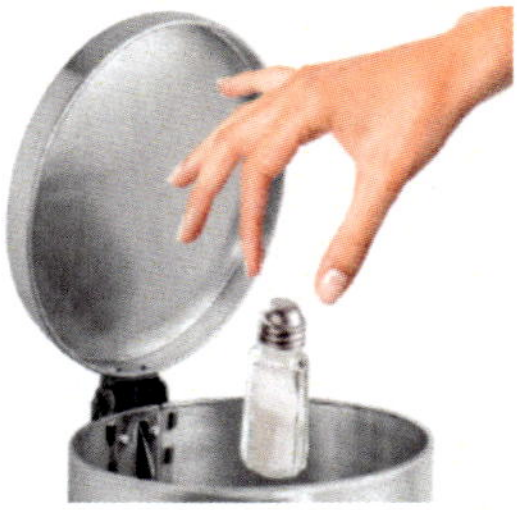

Small, healthy choices can make a huge difference in your life, adding up over time. You can gain traction, get momentum, and ultimately find success in your efforts.

In the long run, any healthy choice is better than an unhealthy one!

TAKE HOME POINTS

Do NOT go on a diet!

Instead, make small healthy choices every day for the rest of your life.

If you have already been committed to diet and exercise and attending to matters of good health, keep it up! Do not feel defeated. CAD can affect people living a healthy lifestyle with no obvious risk factors, implying genetics and unknown other factors at play. If that is your situation, keep up the good work and continue your disciplined approach. Who knows? You might have had to deal with CAD at a much younger age or it might have been even more severe if you had not been making healthy choices.

SO, DOC, HOW BAD IS IT?

If you are facing heart bypass surgery, then you have been diagnosed with CAD. Plaque has built up in your heart arteries forming blockages and impairing blood flow. How much plaque? There are several tools in the modern-day healthcare toolbox useful in evaluating CAD.

Certainly, to begin the evaluation there is no substitute for the familiar "History and Physical" where your doctor can hear about your symptoms and perform an examination of your body. Oftentimes this is only the first step, because findings may be difficult to pick up on, and there may be no indication of CAD based on the discussion and exam alone.

An EKG is performed for almost all patients with a potential cardiac issue; however, even an EKG is not very specific in showing evidence of CAD. An EKG may show evidence of a STEMI or an old heart attack, but in the absence of these findings, an EKG cannot usually determine if a patient has CAD or not. As a result, it is possible for a patient to have severe CAD and a normal EKG.

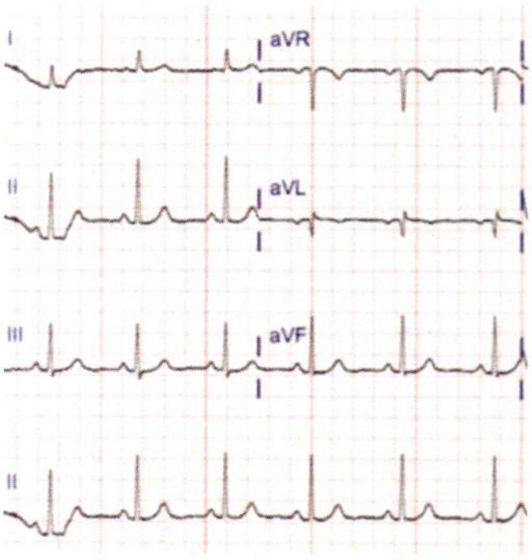

EKG tracing

Another tool helpful in the evaluation of CAD is an echocardiogram, an ultrasound of the heart. A lot of people seem to confuse ElectroCardioGram and Echocardiogram. I think of it like echo goes with sound, such as hearing your voice echo at the Grand Canyon. Electro goes with electricity. An EKG has leads which stick to your chest whereas an Echo has a probe the technician moves around your chest to look at different areas of your heart.

The echo probe sends out a sound wave, the frequency of which is very high and not detectable to the human ear. This ultra-(high)-sound wave bounces off structures of the heart and returns to the probe. The "ultrasound" machine collects the signals and creates images of the heart in motion, allowing evaluation of the heart valves and muscle strength. Views can be assessed from multiple directions, as the technician moves the probe.

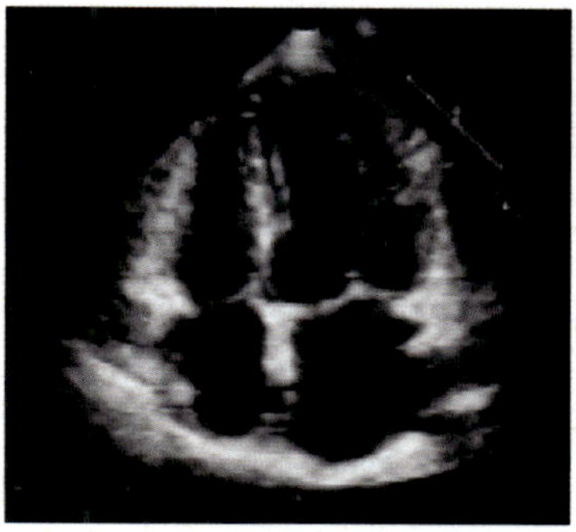

Echo image

There are two main forms of echocardiography: TTE and TEE.

The sound waves of a **Trans Thoracic Echo** (**TTE**) move *trans* the thorax, that is through the chest. The sound waves go through your skin and muscle and bone; these structures can deflect the sound waves, so the technician moves the probe around to get the best images. A TTE is painless, other than mild discomfort which may result from the technician moving the probe around, and usually takes 10-15 minutes.

The sound waves of a **Trans Esophageal Echo** (**TEE**) go *trans* the esophagus, that is through the esophagus. A probe is guided through the mouth into the esophagus, and the sound waves go through the wall of the esophagus. Since the esophagus is directly behind the heart, the probe is closer than with a TTE; plus, skin, muscle and bone are not in the way, resulting in more accurate images of the heart. Typically a mild sedative is given so the patient is not uncomfortable during the procedure, which usually takes about 30 minutes.

For most patients, If a TTE is normal, there is not a reason to do a TEE; but if an abnormality is seen on a TTE, then a TEE may be done to get more information.

Many heart surgeries involve a TEE; that is, a TEE is performed once the patient is asleep in the OR, in order to assess the function of the heart. Also, at the end of the surgery, the TEE helps ensure all valves and all areas of muscle are working well. The TEE provides no useful information while the heart is stopped during an operation.

TAKE HOME POINTS

An Echo uses ultrasound waves to show the heart in motion.

TTE = Trans Thoracic Echo = through the skin

TEE = Trans Esophageal Echo = through the mouth (between the TEEth)

Interestingly, although an echocardiogram provides great information about heart function, it does not actually show blockages of the arteries of the heart. If there has been a bad heart attack with damage to the heart muscle, an echo may show weak muscle contraction. But the actual arteries are not seen and CAD cannot usually be diagnosed from an echo.

How do you know if your heart muscle is strong or weak? Doctors use the term **EF**, which stands for **Ejection Fraction**. The Ejection Fraction is the fraction of blood ejected from the heart with each beat. A normal EF is 60%. When I learned this in medical school it seemed odd to me, because I thought normal would be 100%. But the heart is never empty — it doesn't eject all the blood inside it; in fact, 40% of the blood remains in each chamber after a contraction. This remaining blood ensures no matter how fast the heart beats, it will never be empty.

And the EF is not a matter of personal pride, all you Type-A patients: you don't want it to be 70% or 80%. In fact, an elevated EF of >70%, where the left ventricle appears **hyperdynamic**, often represents the effect of a disease process rather than a strong heart [71]. God made it where 60% is sufficient for effective movement of blood out of the human heart.

Often, a range of values is given by the cardiologist interpreting the echo, rather than a single number.

EJECTION FRACTION	STRENGTH OF HEART MUSCLE
55-60%	Normal
40-45%	Mildly weak
25-30%	Moderately weak
15-20%	Severely weak
5-10%	Profoundly weak

The EF cannot be determined from a physical examination in the doctor's office or an EKG; a TTE or TEE is typically needed to observe the heart muscle in motion to determine the EF.

An EF can be determined for both the left and right ventricles (LVEF and RVEF), though in common usage "EF" by itself refers to the LV.

TAKE HOME POINTS

An EF of 55-60% is normal.

If the EF is low on echo, additional testing is usually needed to determine why the muscle is weak, since the cause could be CAD or something else.

A stress test is an option to assess blood flow to the heart muscle; it shows how well the heart is working when stressed, that is, when it is required to work harder. A stress test can be done with exercise or medications.

An **exercise stress test** involves walking on a treadmill or riding a stationary bicycle. The speed and vigor of the exercise increases as the test goes along. A patient can stop doing the stress test at any time.

Vital signs such as heart rate and blood pressure are monitored during the stress test, as well as an EKG. If any suspicious changes in vital signs or the EKG appear which suggest the heart is struggling, or if the patient experiences chest discomfort, the test is ended.

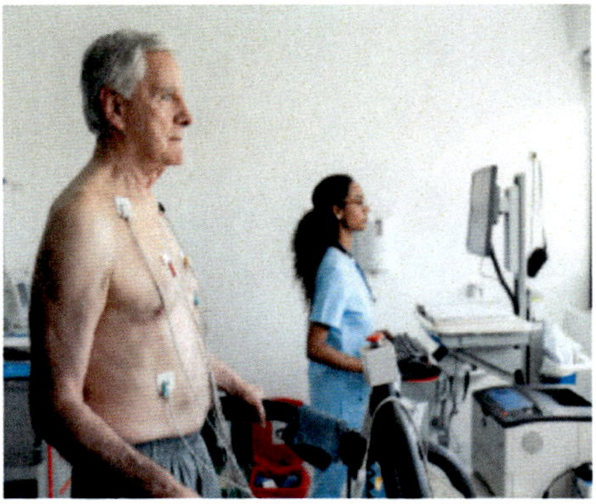

Abnormal findings such as these may be an indicator of CAD and a cardiac catheterization is considered. If the patient completes the test without abnormal findings, then the likelihood of CAD is very low and usually no additional testing is recommended.

A **chemical stress test** can be used instead of the exercise test, for patients who have difficulty walking. A chemical such as dobutamine is given, which increases the heart rate and vigor of myocardial contraction. Vitals and EKG are monitored as with the exercise stress test.

A **nuclear stress test** is another tool that can be used to assess blood flow to the heart. A special chemical known as a radiotracer is injected into a vein. Thallium and sestamibi are common radiotracers. The tracer can be measured with a special detector, both at rest and with exercise. If the patient has a coronary blockage, less blood will flow into the area of the heart served by that coronary artery, and thus the amount of tracer will also be less. Although called "nuclear," the patient is exposed to a tiny amount of radiation with this test — only about 3 times the amount we all encounter in normal day-to-day life.

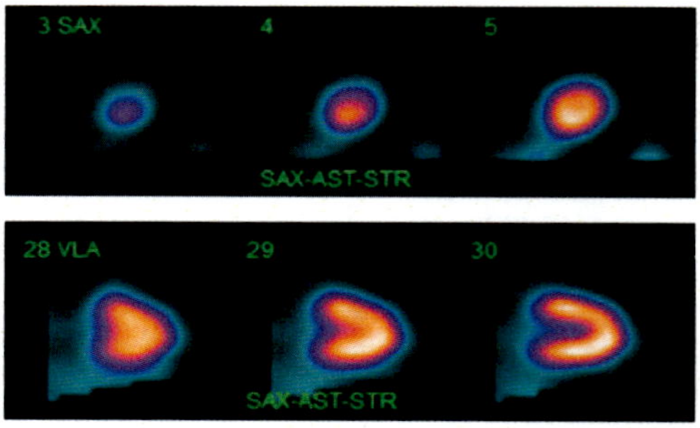

Nuclear stress test images

Keep in mind that a stress test — no matter whether exercise, chemical, or nuclear — does not actually show blockages; rather, it shows evidence of impaired blood flow to heart muscle, which usually only occurs because of blockages. It is possible for blockages to be missed on a stress test. There is no perfect test!

Because of this potential for misleading results, sometimes a cardiologist will recommend a cardiac catheterization even if a stress test is found to be normal, if the cardiologist has a high suspicion of CAD.

When a patient is diagnosed with an NSTEMI, usually a stress test is skipped and a cardiac catheterization is performed, since there is a very high suspicion of CAD. And of course a stress test is skipped in patients with STEMI, because the patient is wheeled into the cath lab at lightning speed — there is no such thing as door-to-treadmill time.

Coronary CTA and **calcium score** are being used more and more as tools in the evaluation of CAD, especially for patients with a low likelihood of CAD. These are often patients who have no symptoms of CAD but have risk factors for it.

Coronary CTA is a special type of CT scan designed to evaluate the coronary arteries for plaque. IV contrast is given for a coronary CTA and both calcified and non-calcified plaque can be visualized. Calcium score evaluates the amount of calcium in the arteries and does not require IV contrast.

Both tests have high accuracy but both tests are generally useful only as screening tests: if a high burden of calcium or plaque is noted on a scan, cardiac catheterization is prudent.

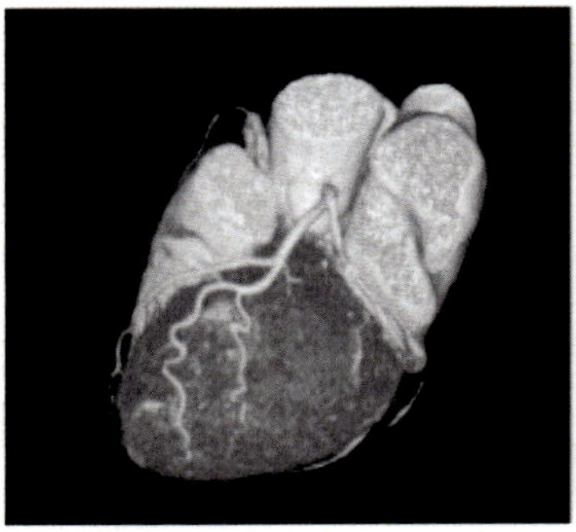

Coronary CTA

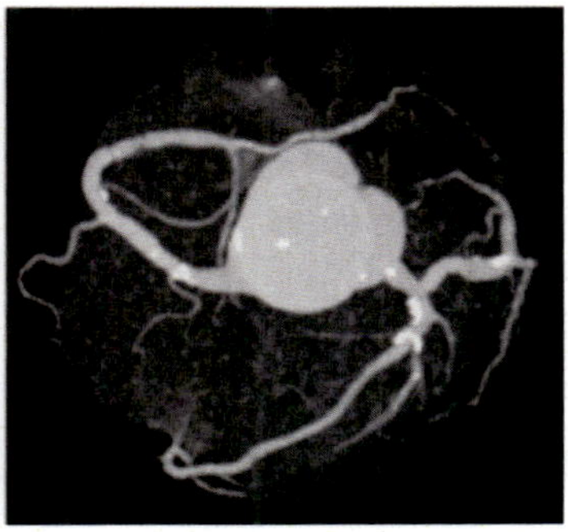

Calcium Score Test

CARDIAC CATHETERIZATION

Cardiac catheterization is the best test to determine the presence of blockages in the coronary arteries. A cardiac catheterization is performed by a heart doctor trained in ways to intervene on the heart – an **interventional cardiologist**. Most doctors call the procedure "cardiac cath" or even just "cath," and a cath is a type of **angiogram**.

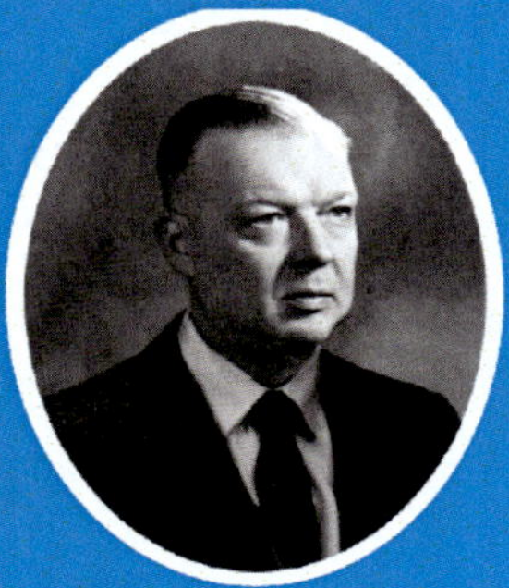

COULD YOU DO THAT?

The **first cardiac cath** in a human was performed in **1929** by **Dr. Werner Forssmann**, a German physician. Twenty-five years old at the time and still in training, he placed a small catheter in a blood vessel in his **own arm** and advanced it into his heart. He then **walked downstairs** and took an x-ray! Although he initially suffered much criticism for his daring act, he received the Nobel Prize in 1956 for his very personal and pioneering work [72].

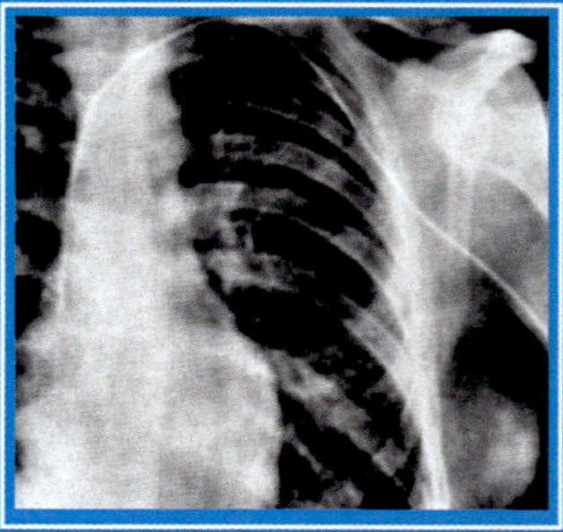

A cath involves numbing the skin near the groin or wrist and puncturing it with a needle. A small plastic tube called a **catheter** is inserted into the artery just beneath the skin and guided into the aorta, then into each coronary artery. Contrast dye is injected, which fills each artery – this particular maneuver is called a **coronary angiogram**. As the contrast dye is injected, a series of x-rays is performed; the x-rays are performed so fast that it looks like a movie showing the arteries filling with the contrast dye. Often, the patient is able to view the images along with the cardiologist, depending on how much sedation has been given.

Occasionally I will read a news headline about a famous person undergoing heart surgery, only to read more details that indicate a cardiac cath was performed. This mixing of nomenclature is confusing, in my opinion; in general, a cardiac cath is a procedure but not surgery. Surgery involves cutting the skin with a scalpel, which is not done with a cardiac cath. A cath is performed by a cardiologist, not a surgeon. Heart surgery is an order of magnitude more complicated than a cardiac cath.

TAKE HOME POINTS

An easy way to offend a heart surgeon is to call him or her a cardiologist.

Wherever the contrast in an artery looks irregular or a segment of artery looks narrowed, plaque in the form of a blockage may be present. If the path of the contrast dye ends abruptly, the artery may be completely blocked. Collateral arteries — the tiny, single-lane channels which connect the major coronaries — can often be seen if a coronary artery has been completely blocked for a while.

A blockage or narrowing — the medical term is **stenosis** — is described by the percent of artery cross-section which is blocked. If half of the cross-section is blocked, the stenosis is 50%. If three-fourths of the cross-section is blocked, the stenosis is 75%. A completely blocked artery has a 100% stenosis, called an **occlusion**.

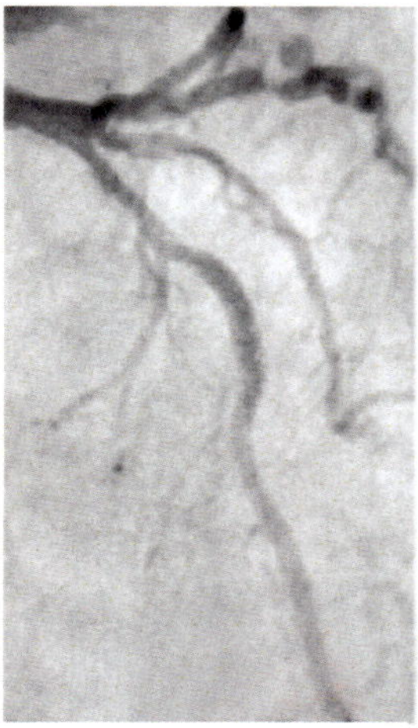

No stenosis

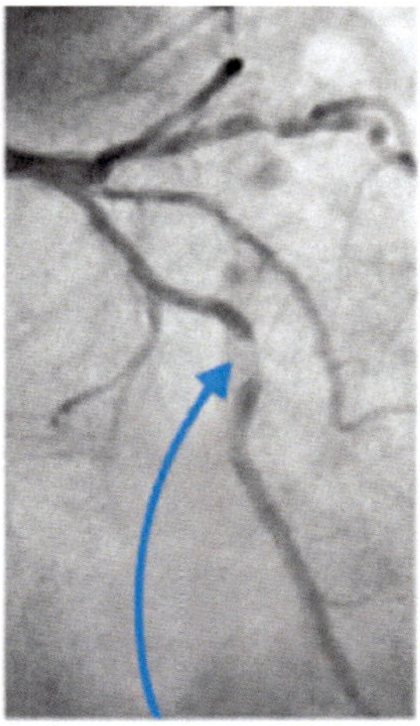

100% occlusion

In a non-diseased state, your coronaries have more capacity for blood flow than you need, even at maximal exercise. This extra capacity allows unimpaired blood flow until a stenosis becomes 60-70%. Blockages less than 60% are concerning, but they can often be treated with medications and without stents or surgery because blood flow is not restricted.

A stenosis greater than 60-70% is more problematic, because blood flow is reduced. In addition, a blockage of 80% or higher often leads to turbulent flow beyond the blockage, as well as a reduction in pressure [74], which decreases the delivery of blood and oxygen.

TAKE HOME POINTS

A significant STENOSIS = a blockage >60-70%.

An OCCLUSION = a 100% blockage.

A stenosis of 80% might possibly be treated with medications alone, if the patient is not having symptoms or weakening of the heart muscle.

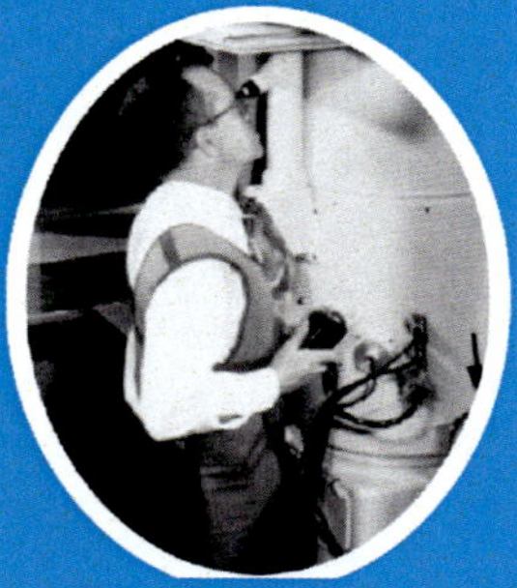

COULD YOU DO THAT?

Nearly 20 years after Dr. Forssmann proved it was safe to insert a catheter into the heart, **Dr. Mason Sones** performed the **first coronary angiogram** at Cleveland Clinic in **1958**.

He did this entirely **by accident.**

When Dr. Sones bent down to view images through a piece of machinery, he instructed his assistant to inject contrast dye, not knowing the catheter had moved into the right coronary artery. He assumed the patient would develop ventricular fibrillation from irritation of the artery, but this did not happen. The event demonstrated that coronary angiography could be performed safely and led to the widespread utilization of the technique [73].

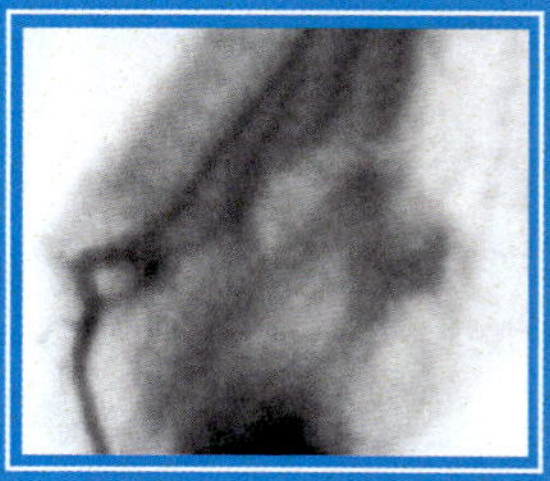

There is no medication that can get rid of the plaque, to melt the blockages away or flatten them out. There is no Drano for the heart. There have been scattered reports of home remedies having such effects but these have not been reproduced in a reliable way in large scientific studies across many programs.

In general, medications are helpful to slow down the process of plaque getting worse, but medications are not effective in getting rid of the plaque. So if a stenosis is already severe and causing symptoms, it will likely need a more aggressive therapy than medications.

One such therapy is **coronary angioplasty**, another procedure performed by an interventional cardiologist. It is also called balloon angioplasty or **PTCA**, short for Percutaneous Transluminal Coronary Angioplasty.

Dr. Andreas Greuntzig in Switzerland performed the first coronary angioplasty in 1977, and around one million angioplasties are now performed in the US each year.

An angioplasty starts the same as a cardiac cath and coronary angiogram, with a puncture of an artery in the groin or wrist and guidance of a catheter into the coronary arteries. The arteries are filled with dye and any stenosis noted. If a significant stenosis is seen, the interventional cardiologist will decide if it can be treated with angioplasty. I think of it as angio**PLA**sty fixes a **PLA**que.

A special tiny balloon is pushed along a tiny wire into the coronary artery and placed within the plaque. The balloon is inflated under great force, pushing the plaque up against the wall of the artery, smushing it and helping to flatten it. This process is ~90% successful in creating more space within the artery for blood to flow[75].

You would think this could cause plaque to break off and block the artery further down-stream but this is not a common problem with the technique.

Patients have asked about the risk of having a stroke due to plaque in a coronary artery breaking off. This is essentially impossible because if any plaque were to break off and move downstream, it would become lodged in a small artery or arteriole of the heart. Plaque cannot move upstream against the flow of the blood, so there is no path coronary plaque could take to get up to the brain.

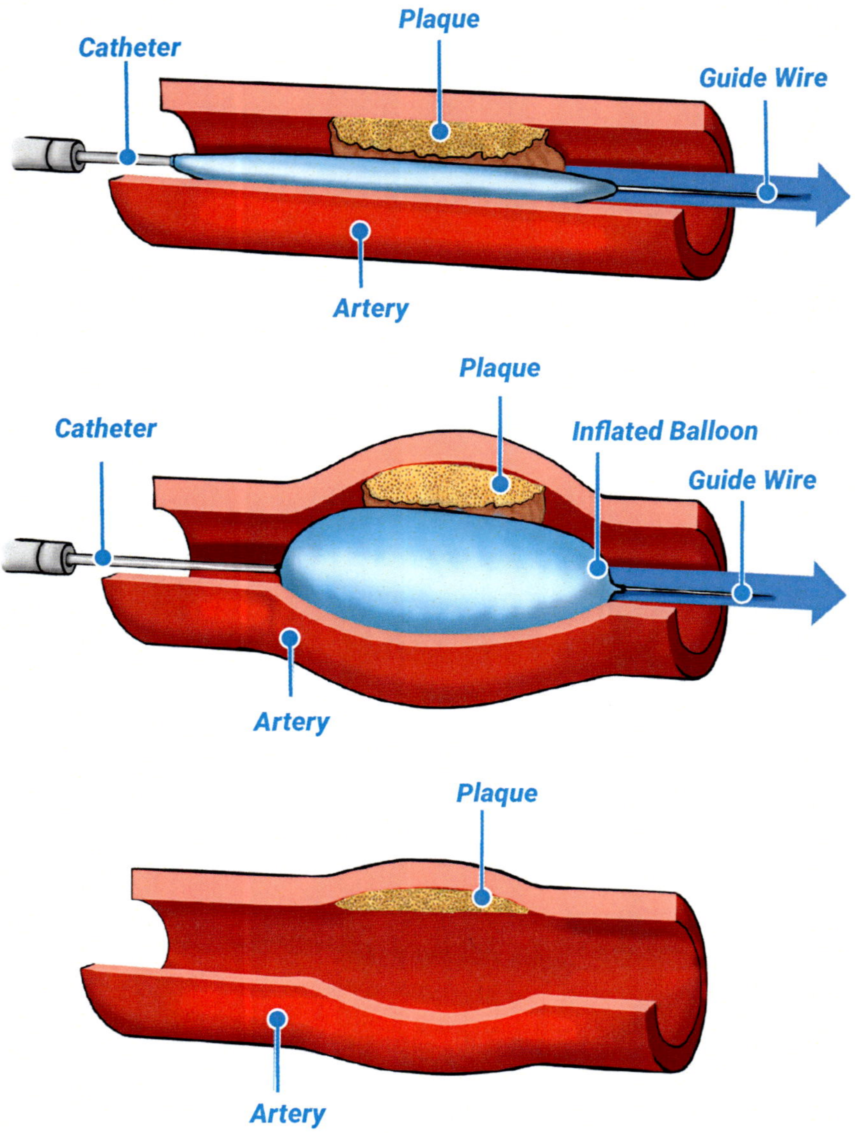

Angioplasty is an appealing technique for treating severe blockages because the trauma to the body is minimal — no incisions are needed, just a puncture. The procedure can take as little as 20-30 minutes and most patients can go home the same day. Complications include injury to an artery such as tearing or rupture, as well as bleeding, but these complications are rare.

The main drawback with angioplasty is impermanence; angioplasty is often highly successful but the effect doesn't last very long. Patients can have blockages worsen again — called **re-stenosis** — and some patients develop new blockages where the balloon was inflated, no doubt due to injury to the endothelium.

TAKE HOME POINTS

Cardiac cath = a catheter goes inside the heart.

Coronary angiogram = contrast dye goes inside the arteries.

Coronary angioPLAsty = a PLAstic balloon goes inside a PLAque.

Coronary stents have been developed to address the issue of re-stenosis and provide a more durable option over angioplasty. A **stent** is a small metal tube used to hold open the artery/plaque.

The process of placing a stent is called **PCI**, Percutaneous Coronary Intervention. It starts off like a cath, with a puncture in the groin or wrist, manipulation of the catheter into the coronaries, and determination of the location of the stenosis. PCI is performed by... guess who? An interventional cardiologist.

EXTRA CREDIT

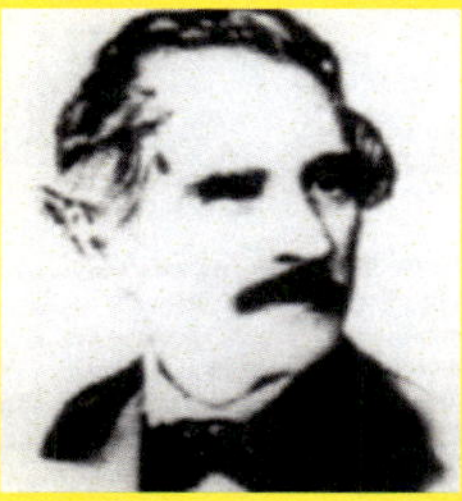

The term "stent" comes from the name of **Charles Thomas Stent**, an English dentist. In the mid 1800s, he developed a compound to set dentures, based on a natural latex called Gutta-percha produced by tropical trees [76]. Dr. Johannes Esser, a Dutch plastic surgeon, later used the compound to stabilize skin grafts, detailing its merits in his book *Plastic Surgery of the Face*. The term gained popularity and continued in common usage, even after the compound fell out of favor.

There are different sizes and lengths of stents; the appropriate stent is chosen by the interventional cardiologist based on the features of the artery and the stenosis. Sometimes more than one stent is needed to treat a particular stenosis. The stent is loaded onto a balloon in a compressed state, smaller than the final shape. The stent-on-balloon is guided along a wire into position within the stenosis. The live x-ray shows the position and the balloon is inflated, as with angioplasty, smushing the plaque to the sides.

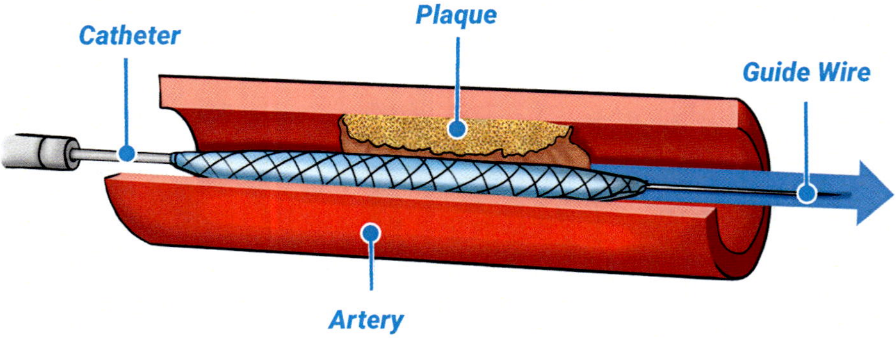

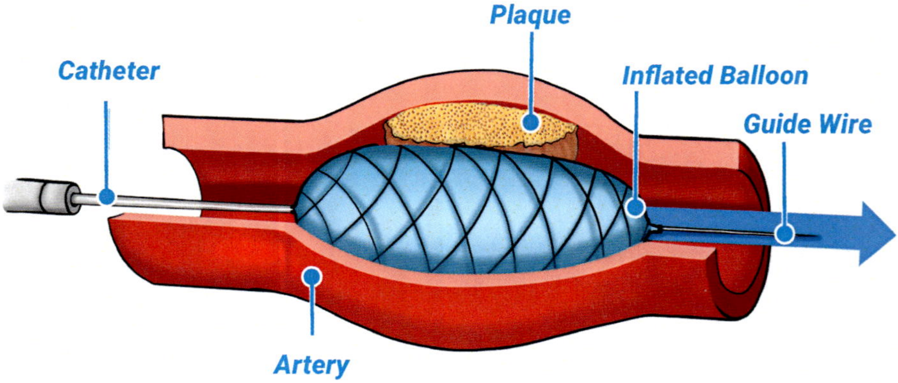

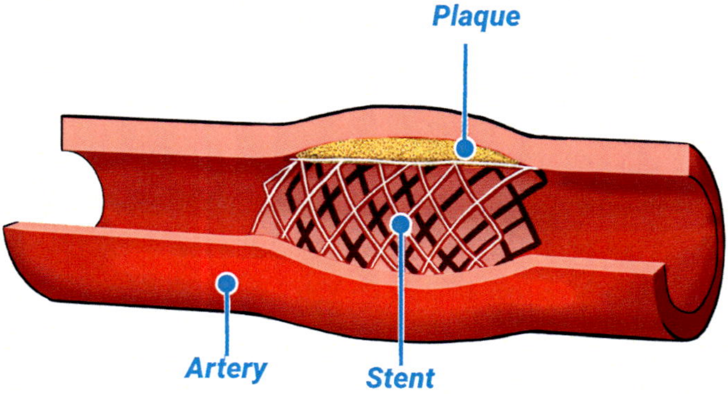

The stent is opened by the balloon and takes its permanent shape as a hollow tube, holding open the plaque and artery. The balloon and wire are removed, while the outward force of the stent against the artery wall and plaque keeps the stent in position.

PCI is an excellent option for many patients with CAD. If a patient only has one blockage, the interventional cardiologist will likely place a stent. However, if the Left Main coronary is tightly blocked or if all three coronary arteries have blockages, then bypass surgery is usually recommended instead of stents.

This recommendation is particularly strong for diabetic patients.

Sometimes, due to heavy calcification or tight angulation of an artery, even a single stenosis cannot be stented and bypass surgery is needed.

Most patients can go home the same day or the next day after PCI. Patients may have some soreness at the site of puncture (groin or wrist), but generally get back to normal day-to-day activity within a couple of days.

STENT-OLOGY

The first stent was placed in 1986, a type of stent known as **a bare-metal stent** (**BMS**). It looks like a tube made of very fine chicken wire, only stronger. Bare-metal stents were found to be better than angioplasty in terms of avoiding re-stenosis, but the results were still not ideal.

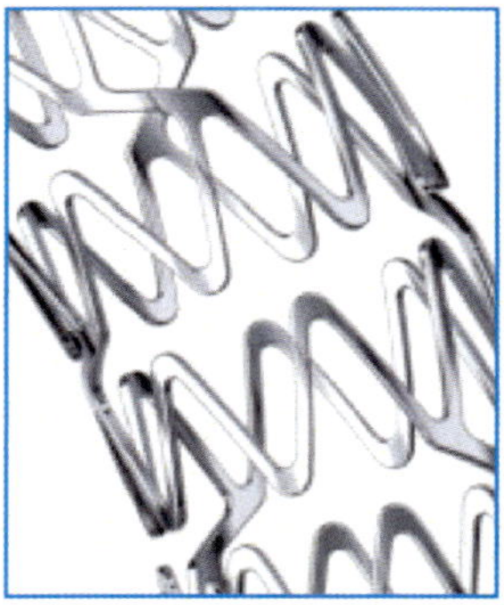

Close-up of Bare Metal Stent

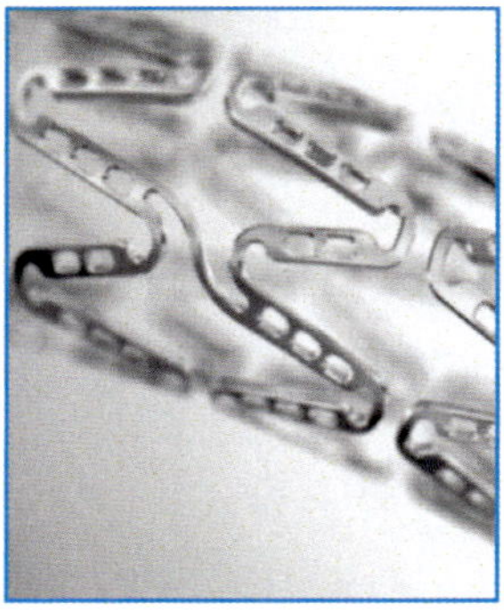

Close-up of Drug-Eluting Stent

In 1999, the first **drug-eluting stent** (**DES**) was placed. A drug-eluting stent elutes a drug, meaning that it releases a drug. The metal frame is coated with a thin polymer that releases a drug in tiny amounts. The drug is designed to decrease the overgrowth of cells and discourage the attachment of platelets within the stent.

The frame of the first stents was made of stainless steel. Many current stents are made of a cobalt-chromium alloy, which can be made with a thinner profile yet maintain adequate strength. More recently, a few platinum-chromium alloy stents have been released on the market; they are priced like they are made of platinum and vibranium!

Actually, the ballpark cost to a hospital for a DES is around $2,500 (prices are all over the map depending on hospital contracts), which is not too bad given the complexity of the technology, in my opinion.

Every commercially available stent is man-made and foreign to the human body. All of your blood vessels are lined with endothelial cells unique to you, as you know from your diligent reading. Your blood happily flows when in contact with your endothelium but clots when it touches anything else. Any non-endothelial material — such as proteins hidden inside a plaque or the surface of a metal object — will quickly cause a clotting reaction, starting with platelets.

When a stent is placed inside a coronary artery, platelets passing through the stent will stick to the stent. If a lot of platelets stick and if the platelets start to stick to each other, the entire stent can become blocked, which is called **stent thrombosis**. Stent thrombosis can cause a heart attack and even death. Fortunately, stent thrombosis is uncommon, complicating only about 1-2% of bare metal stents and 0.5% of DES [77].

Could stents be coated with endothelium from your body, in order to reduce the risk of thrombosis? Could your endothelial cells be grown in a lab and used like paint to coat the inside of a stent? While no such option currently exists, such a biologically engineered solution would be a leap forward in stent technology.

PICK YOUR POISON

In order to minimize the risk of stent thrombosis, a patient with a new stent is treated with **DAPT**, aka **Dual Anti-Platelet Therapy**. Aspirin and Plavix are a common combination used for DAPT. Any medicine in the same class as Plavix — which is an ADP/P2Y receptor inhibitor, for all you pharmacology trivia buffs – can also be used; Effient and Brilinta are examples.

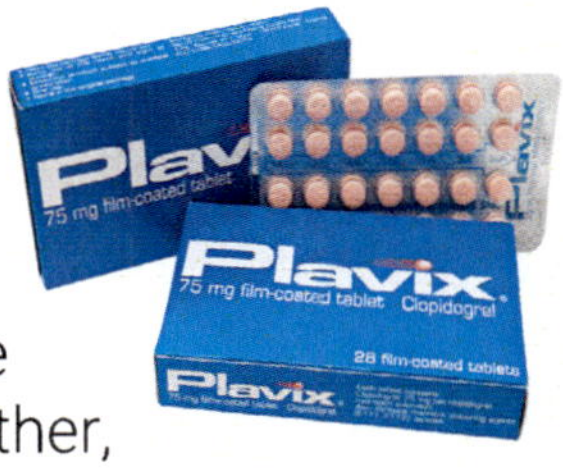

Aspirin reduces platelet clumping by stopping one of the chemicals platelets use to attach to each other, **cyclo-oxygenase** (**COX**). Plavix works by binding the P2Y receptor on platelets, causing each platelet to be less likely to bind to another platelet.

When a patient is on both Aspirin and Plavix, the platelets are affected in two different ways and platelet function is reduced a lot, significantly lowering the risk of stent thrombosis.

However, since the platelets do not bind together very well, the flip side of DAPT is a higher risk of bleeding. Some patients report excessive bruising, where minor bumps or falls lead to larger-than-expected bruises or injuries. If a patient has a bleeding stomach ulcer, it may bleed more than it would have if the patient were not on Aspirin and Plavix.

If significant bleeding occurs, Plavix will usually need to be stopped; this is true for patients needing surgery as well. Plavix does not tend to *cause* bleeding, but it can make bleeding worse when it happens.

For a new stent, Plavix is needed until the body coats the inside of the stent with endothelium. After a layer of endothelial cells completely coats the inside of the stent, platelets do not distinguish the stent from a normal blood vessel and will not stick to the stent. At that point, the risk of stent thrombosis is low, so Plavix can often be stopped.

Typically, Aspirin is continued, and for most patients Aspirin is not stopped except for a compelling reason (cardiologists love Aspirin – I'm suspicious they have put it in the water supply but haven't told the rest of us).

With a bare-metal stent, the endothelium lining usually takes 3-6 months to form, so Plavix can be stopped after 6 months. With drug-eluting stents, the time is longer. This seems backwards because the drug eluted by the stent itself is supposed to keep the stent from getting clogged, right? The reason is the drug released by the stent is designed to slow the growth of cells inside the stent.

I think of it like the drug is stopping scar tissue from forming inside the stent. But the drug released by the stent does not inhibit platelets all that much, so Aspirin and Plavix are still needed. In addition, since the drug slows the growth of cells— which is good for stopping scar formation — it also slows down the lining of the stent with endothelial cells. Thus, it takes longer for the endothelium to form inside a DES, 12 months rather than 6; so Plavix is needed for 12 months, and then Plavix can usually be safely stopped.

In everyday life, a cardiologist may keep a patient on Plavix for much longer, sometimes never stopping the Plavix.

TAKE HOME POINTS

Bare Metal Stents & Drug-Eluting Stents are placed via PCI.

Stents require Dual Anti-Platelet Therapy, such as Aspirin & Plavix:

BMS = 3-6 months vs. DES = 12 months

Aspirin is generally taken daily either as a full dose of 325mg or as a “baby” dose of 81mg. Although many doctors prescribe Aspirin to any older patient, recent evidence has called this practice into question [78], and many older patients probably do not need to take Aspirin. For patients who have had a heart attack or stroke, low-dose Aspirin may be beneficial. It is best to discuss the particulars of Aspirin therapy with your cardiologist. Ask how much they put in the drinking water while you’re there!

In general, a “baby Aspirin” is sufficient to reduce platelet clumping and the full dose of 325 mg does not provide much additional benefit. Since a full dose of Aspirin can be associated with a higher risk of bleeding than the lower dose, I usually prefer for my bypass surgery patients to only take a daily baby Aspirin prior to operation. It can be taken up to the night before the operation. Unless there is an emergency, Plavix needs to be stopped prior to operation; otherwise, Plavix raises the risk of excessive bleeding after the operation.

There is no antidote to Plavix; that is, there is not another medicine that can be given to counteract its effect. Another way to put it is that Plavix has an irreversible effect on platelets – once it binds to a platelet, it cannot be unbound. So if bleeding occurs during surgery, the only option is to transfuse platelets from another person (who was not on Plavix). Then the transfused platelets will clump and the bleeding will stop.

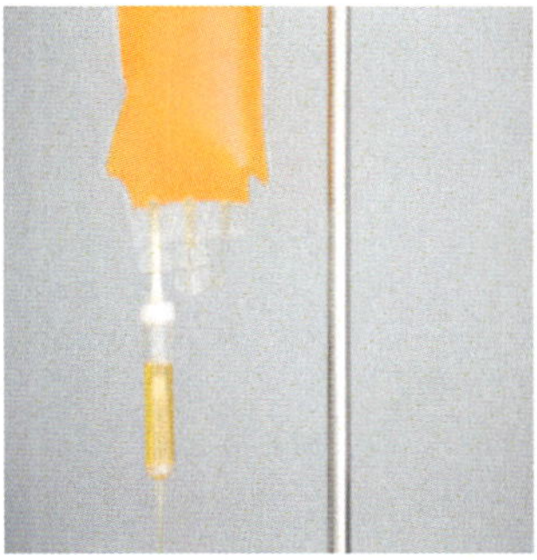

Bag of platelets for transfusion

However, it is preferable not to transfuse any blood component from another person, if possible. The better option is to stop Plavix prior to operation and allow time for new platelets to be made by the body. The new platelets will not be affected by Plavix. It usually takes 7 days to replace all of your platelets with new ones, so we **stop Plavix for 7 days** prior to surgery. If a patient has a fresh stent, we usually admit the patient to the hospital several days prior to bypass surgery and switch to a different medicine given IV which has a reversible effect, unlike Plavix.

If a patient undergoes bypass surgery but did not have a heart attack, I usually send the patient home on Aspirin without any Plavix. The reason is that no foreign material is exposed to the bloodstream with surgery: there are no stents, and the bypass grafts are native to the patient. So the patient's endothelium is coating the inside of every vessel already such that there is a low risk of thrombosis. Thus, no Plavix is needed.

In cases of bypass surgery performed after a heart attack, we usually send a patient home on Plavix for 3-6 months, as this has been declared desirable by national groups such as the American Heart Association. Still, the decision is made on a case-by-case basis, taking the risks and benefits for each patient into account.

CORONARY ANATOMY

The heart is easy to understand provided you don't look at it.
John Glynn [18]

The heart is able to convert chemical energy from food into mechanical energy to pump blood. Try figuring out how to do that! This remarkable process requires oxygen. You might assume the oxygen in the blood can simply diffuse (move) from inside the heart into the muscle, but you are not a jellyfish and the muscle is too thick for this to happen. The heart muscle needs its own oxygen and its own blood supply. The **coronary arteries** provide blood to the heart muscle, which as you know is called myocardium.

The heart is unique in that it is the only organ which provides its own blood flow; it pumps its own blood through the coronary arteries and coronary veins, which form the 3rd circulation of the human body. It takes blood only 1-2 seconds to complete the coronary circulation [18].

Coronary comes from *corona*, the Latin word for crown, because to early anatomists, the arteries of the heart looked like a crown. Perhaps they were subconsciously acknowledging the heart as king of the body organs.

The heart is not like most organs where the major arteries are located deep within the organ, such as the brain, lungs, kidneys, and liver. The heart is a super-organ, remember? Instead of being inside, the arteries of the heart are located on the surface. This is pertinent to bypass surgery because the heart does not need to be opened to perform bypasses. Bypass surgery is often called open-heart surgery, but technically the heart itself is not opened in the sense that the surgeon is not looking at or working on the inside of the heart.

Another interesting aspect of the coronary arteries is that most of the blood flow within the coronaries occurs during diastole, when the myocardium relaxes and the ventricles fill. This is unusual because most other branches of the aorta deliver blood during systole. Blood moves into your brain and other organs when the heart contracts, but blood moves into your heart muscle when it relaxes. About 80% of the blood moves during diastole and 20% during systole [79].

TAKE HOME POINTS

The coronary arteries are on the outside of the heart & fill with blood when the heart relaxes.

The coronaries are the first branches of the aorta, arising just above the aortic valve; almost as soon as blood exits the heart through the aortic valve, some of the blood enters the coronary arteries. About 5% of the blood pumped out of your heart goes into the coronaries in a resting state. This amount is 10 times as much per gram of tissue than the rest of the body as a whole, [79] indicative of the high metabolic demand of the heart.

The two coronaries which arise from the aorta just above the valve are the Left Main Coronary Artery and the Right Coronary Artery.

The Left Main Coronary Artery is often called simply the "**Left Main**." After a short distance, the Left Main splits into the LAD and the (Left) Circumflex artery. Because the Left Main supplies almost all of the blood flow to the left side of the heart — which as you know performs considerably more work than the right side — blockages in the Left Main can be particularly dangerous.

The term **LAD** — pronounced "L.A.D." — is shorthand for Left Anterior Descending. As a matter of practical usage, no one ever says the "LAD artery" or the "Left Anterior Descending artery" — it's just called the LAD. The LAD starts as a branch of the Left Main and serves the **L**eft ventricle, it courses on the front or **A**nterior part of the heart, and it courses from the top of the heart to the bottom (**D**escending).

The LAD is colloquially called the "widowmaker," because it provides so much of the blood to the left ventricle that a heart attack involving the LAD can be life-threatening.

Although the LAD and Circumflex are the two branches of the Left Main, they are not of equal importance — the Circumflex is not called widowmaker #2 or anything like that.

The Left **Circumflex** artery is often simply called the "Circumflex," abbreviated as "Cx." It serves some of the left side and back of the heart.

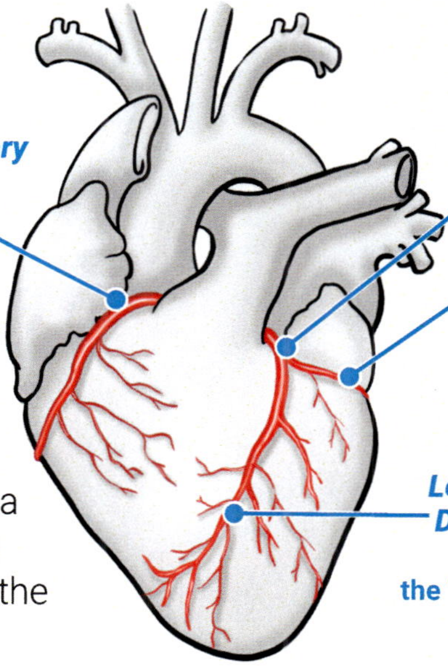

The **Right Coronary Artery** is often called simply "the Right" or "R.C.A." It branches directly off the aorta and serves the right side of the heart and some of the back of the heart.

Since the right ventricle does not perform as much work as the LV, the RCA is considered slightly less important than the LAD or Circumflex. Indeed, blockages of the RCA often cause less symptoms than similar blockages of the LAD or Circumflex and may even be asymptomatic. Still, you can never quite predict what will happen because in some other cases the RCA may cause big problems!

TAKE HOME POINTS

The Left Main & RCA arise from the aorta.

The Left Main branches into the LAD & Circumflex.

In the game of coronary chess, the Left Main is KING & the LAD is QUEEN.

The coronary arteries have branches. And branches of branches. All 3 circulatory systems (pulmonary, systemic, coronary) are designed with arteries that branch many times. These branches give rise to **arterioles** and then **capillaries** where gas exchange occurs. Then venules take over, leading to veins which get larger and larger until blood returns to the heart. Whew — to go through all of that feels like work! Indeed, it is estimated that every red blood cell in your blood travels 12,000 miles each day, traversing your circulatory system over and over and over again [18].

Some common, sizeable branches of the major coronary arteries are:

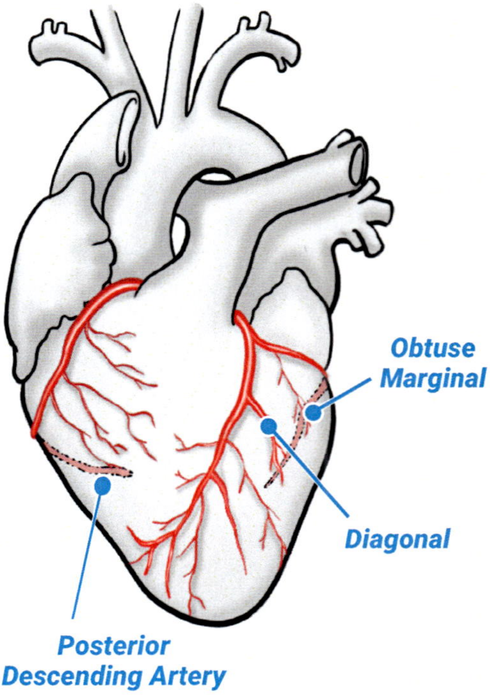

Diagonal: branch of the LAD, on the front of the heart.

OM: aka Obtuse Marginal; branch of the Circumflex, on the left side of the heart.

PDA: aka Posterior Descending Artery; a branch of the RCA or sometimes the Circumflex, on the back of the heart.

Ramus: aka Ramus Intermedius; a branch of the Left Main which occurs in ~30% of patients [80].

The branches can sometimes be even more complicated: If there are multiple sizeable branches from one of the major coronaries (LAD, Cx, RCA), then the branches have numbers.

For example, if two diagonals arise from the LAD, the first is described as D1 and the second is D2. It is fairly common for a patient to have two OMs arising from the Circumflex.

For some patients, the coronary artery branches are quite small, too small for stents or bypass grafts when affected by CAD. For other patients, a branch may be quite large. In some cases, a branch may even rival one of the major coronaries in size.

EXTRA CREDIT

The intricate branching pattern of arteries and veins is similar to the bronchial tree in the lungs, as well as the branching pattern of trees and coral. These shared patterns are based on fractals, a mathematical concept also found in lightning, snowflakes, waterfalls, canyons, coastlines, electricity and indeed almost all of nature.

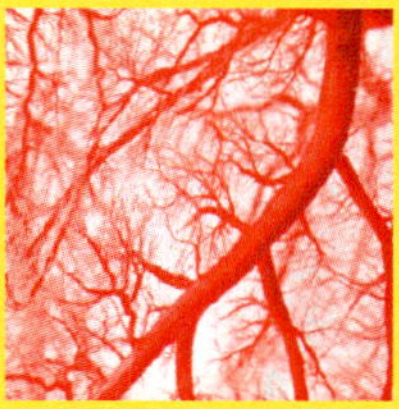
Arteries

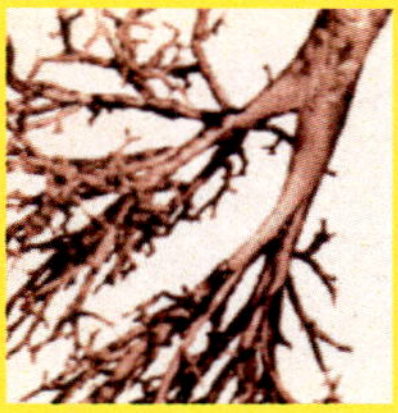
Bronchi

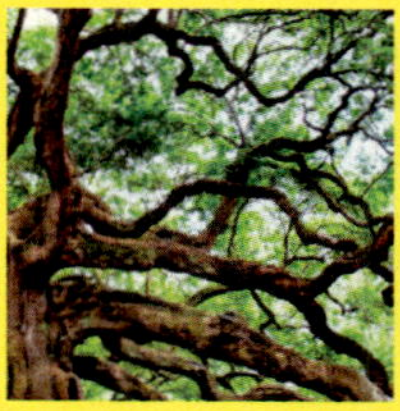
Trees

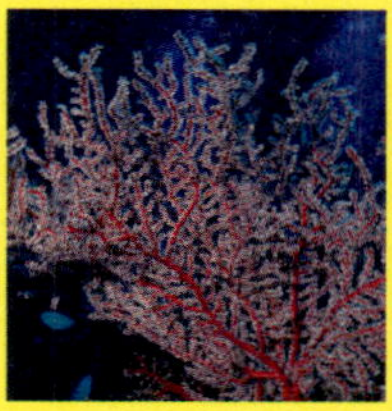
Coral

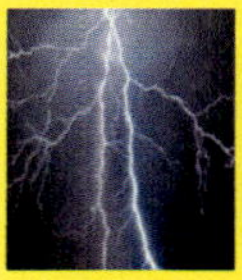
Lightning

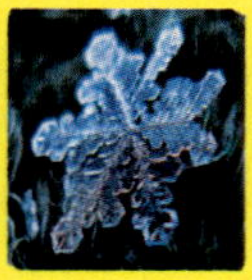
Snowflake

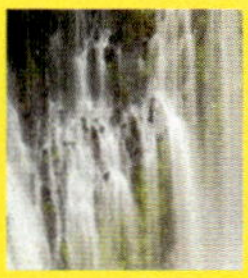
Waterfall

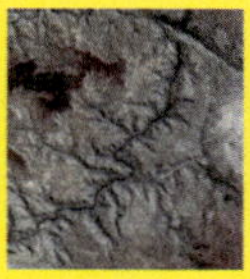
Grand Canyon

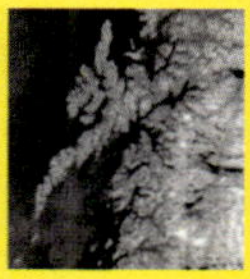
Coastline

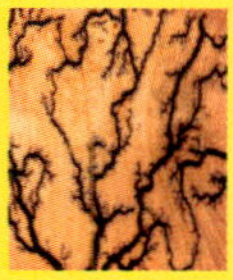
Wood-Burning

Some people might interpret these shared features to be a matter of evolutionary physics, but I take it to mean God has a preference on how He designs things!

CAD can affect one, two or all three of the major coronary arteries, as well as the branches.

Once CAD is identified on cath, a decision can be made regarding therapy, on a case by case basis. Options typically include medications, stent(s), and bypass surgery.

TAKE HOME POINTS

The LAD often has a Diagonal branch, sometimes two.

The Circumflex often has two branches, OM1 & OM2.

The RCA often has a PDA branch.

The Left Main has a extra branch called the Ramus in 30% of patients.

WHEN A SURGEON IS NEEDED

You can't always get what you want,
But if you try, sometime you find
You get what you need.
Mick Jagger and Keith Richards [81]

If all other factors were equal, almost everyone would pick a stent over surgery; the procedure is shorter, the stay in hospital is less and the recovery is quicker for most patients with a stent.

But all other factors are not equal. Bypass surgery has been found to be a superior option in many cases, such as:

Left Main stenosis. It can be treacherous to place a stent in the Left Main because flow to the LAD or Circumflex can accidentally be compromised. Bypass surgery is recommended for most of these patients.

Triple-vessel disease. If the LAD, Cx and RCA all have severe blockages, studies have shown diabetic patients will live longer (statistically-speaking) with bypass surgery instead of stents. The data is so compelling for diabetic patients that bypass is offered to many patients with triple-vessel disease, even if not diabetic.

A non-stentable stenosis, aka a blockage which cannot be fixed with a stent. A stenosis in a heavily-calcified artery or in a sharply-angled section of an artery often cannot be safely stented. Similarly, a stenosis of 100% (an occlusion) often cannot be opened with a stent, or at least the process to try to stent an occlusion can be treacherous.

Re-stenosis. Bypass surgery is often considered after a stent has already been placed and failed to stay open, particularly if the re-stenosis occurred soon after stent placement.

There are many other scenarios where bypass surgery may be considered. The decision of figuring out the best option among medications, stents, or bypass surgery is made on an individualized basis. The decision is ultimately yours. Your cardiologist and surgeon will provide information and support to help you in decision-making.

CHOOSING A SURGEON

There are roughly 4,000 **cardiothoracic (CT) surgeons** in the USA. Some surgeons perform only cardiac (heart) surgery, some only thoracic (lung) surgery and some perform both.

Finding the right surgeon can be an intimidating task. Most patients simply go with the surgeon suggested by their cardiologist, trusting the cardiologist's recommendation.

In a small town, there may only be one CT surgeon and you may not feel like you have much of a choice. Larger cities will have many surgeons and many facilities. If your situation is not an emergency, it is worth discussing with friends and family whether travelling to a larger city or seeking out a large program may be worth it for you.

The **American Board of Thoracic Surgery** (**ABTS**) provides Board certification for cardiothoracic surgeons in the USA. Barring an emergency situation, there is no compelling reason to settle for a surgeon who is not Board-certified. You should insist on having a Board-certified surgeon!

Board certification cannot ensure a surgeon is excellent or outstanding, but it does indicate the surgeon has passed the testing needed to prove competency in heart surgery. If a surgeon is not Board-certified, it means he or she has recently completed training (and has limited experience) and/or has not successfully passed the testing/certification process.

TAKE HOME POINTS

Find a Board-certified surgeon.

In addition to Board certification, it is reasonable and prudent to ask your surgeon how many bypass operations he or she has performed. You may also want to ask how many bypass surgeries the surgeon performs per year.

There may not be a magic number which will make or break the deal, but generally the greater the number of surgeries, the more experience the surgeon has. Some groups have suggested an expert (high-volume) surgeon will likely perform at least 100 bypass operations per year [82].

Plan to ask about your surgeon's outcomes after bypass surgery, such as the rate of death, stroke, or other complications. The rates of complications will depend on patient risk factors (some surgeons are willing to operate on high-risk patients and some are not), but rates of death and stroke can generally be expected to be in the 1-2% range.

You can ask the same questions about the facility in which you will have your operation.

Ask as many questions as it takes to be comfortable with your understanding of your operation, your surgeon and the facility. Do not ever feel bad about asking questions!

TAKE HOME POINTS

Never hesitate to ask questions.

It is notoriously difficult for the public to gauge the level of quality of a doctor or surgeon. There are some helpful websites such as:

www.ratemds.com **www.healthgrades.com**

www.webmd.com **www.vitals.com**

These sites may be better than nothing but can be skewed by extremely happy or unhappy patients, and oftentimes the reviews are mostly an indicator of how the patient *felt* the surgeon treated them and not an indicator of how skilled the surgeon may be in performing an operation.

A friend-of-a-friend reference is much better, especially for those with connections to the healthcare community. You can also ask nurses and staff at the hospital their opinion about your surgeon.

Beyond an objective "data-style" aspect of choosing a good surgeon, there is a subjective "how-do-you-feel" aspect. Consider how you feel when you speak with your surgeon. If you feel respected and feel your surgeon cares about you, go for it! If not, do not be afraid to recognize your reservations. Don't feel bad if you just don't like your surgeon (or any doctor). Sometimes people – even two "great" people – may not hit it off for some reason; same is true of surgeon and patient.

Your level of comfort with your surgeon is key to your care. If your surgeon is Board-certified, performs a reasonable number of bypass surgeries every year with good outcomes, and has gained your confidence in consultation, you will be primed for success; your surgeon will be hard to beat.

If your surgeon is not Board-certified, has a low volume practice or poor outcomes, and/or did not gain your confidence in consultation, then you may want to think twice before proceeding. You will likely benefit from a **second opinion**.

Certainly, if the surgeon is any way rude or dismissive, find another one! Gone are the days when a surgeon could be rude but still have a large practice, with people putting up with a horrid bedside manner thinking it was "worth it." We live in a social media-connected, review-savvy world, and poor customer service doesn't cut it these days, even in healthcare. Feeling disrespected is not worth it, and you can expect to be treated with dignity and respect at all times by your surgeon. Do not settle for less.

Seeking a second opinion seems to be an underused approach — many patients do not seek a second opinion. Now, I don't know about you, but if I need the foundation of my house fixed, I'm getting several quotes! A lot of people do. But not with heart surgery? Seems odd to me, since your heart is surely more precious than your house.

Of course it is not wrong to go with the surgeon you first meet, but if you have *any* reservations, by all means get a second opinion. Or even a third.

Some patients seem to think it may offend the surgeon or be awkward to ask, but as a professional I can assure you, there is nothing awkward about it. There is absolutely nothing wrong with asking for a second opinion. If nothing else, a second opinion will likely provide additional peace of mind and give you confidence in your surgical path.

If you would like to seek a second opinion, let your cardiologist or surgeon know and ask for another surgeon's name and contact info. Almost all doctors will be happy to help.

If a doctor or surgeon becomes upset at your asking for a second opinion, then that is not a doctor I would recommend continuing to see, because the person's ego is interfering with their ability to meet your needs.

TAKE HOME POINTS

Never hesitate to get a second opinion.

HOW BYPASS IS DONE

I chose the road less traveled and now I don't know where I am.
Anonymous

Heart bypass surgery has been performed millions of times over the past few decades and has been honed into a reproducible, effective operation. It is a well-worn path, and following that pathway leads to reliable results.

The core concept with bypass surgery is creation of a new pathway added to the coronary circulation through which blood can flow and deliver oxygen to the myocardium. Instead of "heart bypass surgery," at the hospital we call it **CABG**, pronounced "Cabbage," which stands for Coronary Artery Bypass Grafting.

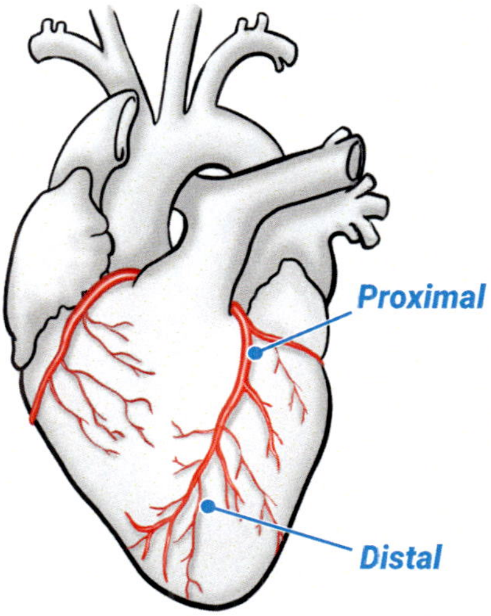

An interesting quirk of CAD is that most blockages occur in a **proximal** segment of a coronary artery, that is, not far from where the artery begins. This is in contrast to a **distal** segment further away from the artery's origin. For example, most blockages of the RCA occur in the proximal half of the artery [83].

Another way to phrase it is past the blockage, the rest of an artery often isn't too bad. Of course there are exceptions, but this pattern of disease allows CABG to be a great option for many patients.

With CABG, the blockages in the coronaries are not usually modified, meaning the surgeon does not remove the blockages, stent them, or even touch them. Instead, the surgeon goes past each blockage and adds a new pathway for blood to flow to the heart muscle around the blockage.

The new pathway is called a **bypass graft** and the vessel used is the **conduit**. I think of conduit like biological tubing; it must be biological because plastic tubing doesn't work — plastic was tried once upon a time but it easily became blocked with blood clots (thrombus). Surgeons have also tried veins from cows (bovine) and the human umbilical cord, but these don't stay open very long either.

The best conduit to use is a blood vessel from the patient's own body, often an artery and a vein. Which conduit is used for your operation in particular will depend on your anatomy and the surgical plan to address the blockages. The process used to prepare a conduit during the operation is called the **harvest**.

For almost all patients, the **LIMA** is used — pronounced "LEE-ma." LIMA is short for Left Internal Mammary Artery, which is the artery located next to your breastbone on the left side. It provides blood to the tissues of your chest wall. It works great as a conduit because it is roughly the same size as the coronary arteries and has great blood flow.

EXTRA CREDIT

In 1950, Dr. Vineberg became the first surgeon to use the LIMA in the treatment of heart disease. He created a tunnel in the heart muscle and sewed the end of the LIMA into the muscle, not connecting it to a coronary artery.

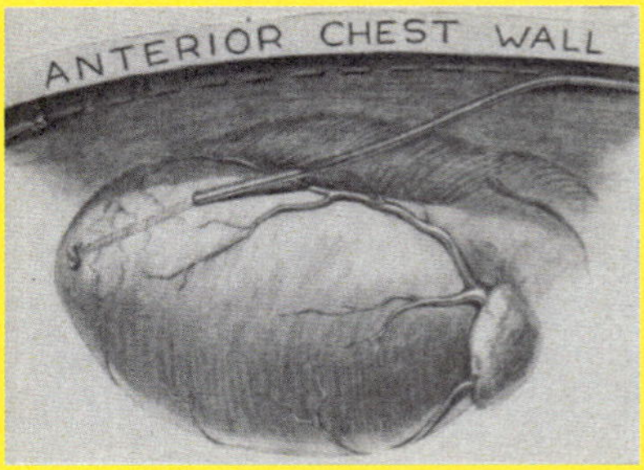

Tunneled LIMA, part of Vineberg Operation [85]

His patients did very well but other surgeons had difficulty reproducing his excellent results. In time, the modern technique of CABG with connection of the LIMA to the LAD was developed and the Vineberg Operation was relegated to the history books.

The LIMA has great blood flow because it almost never has its own blockages; this is because the LIMA has a specialized endothelium which produces **nitric oxide**, the equivalent of releasing tiny doses of nitroglycerin into the artery all the time [84].

Your ribs provide blood to the same tissues of the chest wall such that the chest wall is not damaged when the LIMA is diverted and used as a conduit for bypass grafting.

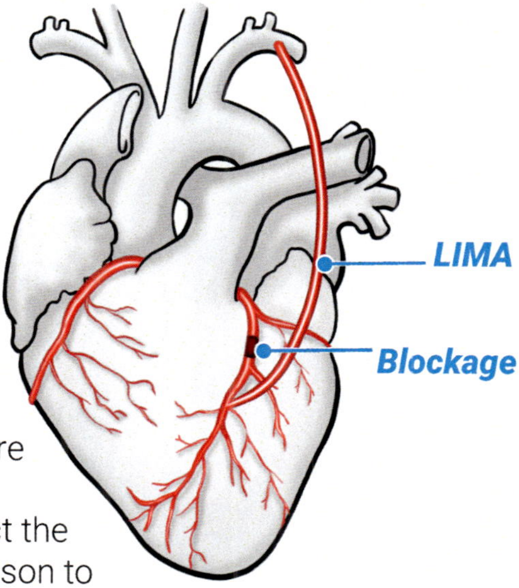

During CABG, the distal (far) end of the LIMA is separated from the surrounding tissues, near the bottom of your ribcage; this allows the end of the LIMA to swing down and attach to the LAD.

The proximal end of the LIMA, where it arises from the subclavian artery near your collarbone, remains intact the way God made it, as there is no reason to disconnect it on that end.

The LIMA is almost always used to graft the LAD, unless there is a compelling reason not to, because this has been found to be the most effective bypass graft combination.

The LIMA and the LAD are connected using a tiny needle and suture, sewn by hand. The suture is a blue monofilament thread, like very thin fishing line; it is roughly the same size and strength as a human hair. The connection created between the two arteries is called an **anastomosis**.

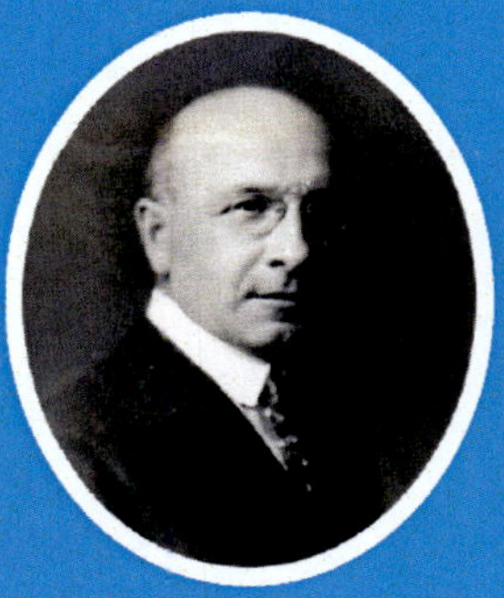

COULD YOU DO THAT?

French surgeon **Alexis Carrel** perfected the method of connecting two blood vessels together in an **anastomosis**. He received the Nobel Prize in **1912** for his work [86]. The basic method he developed is **still being used** over 100 years later!

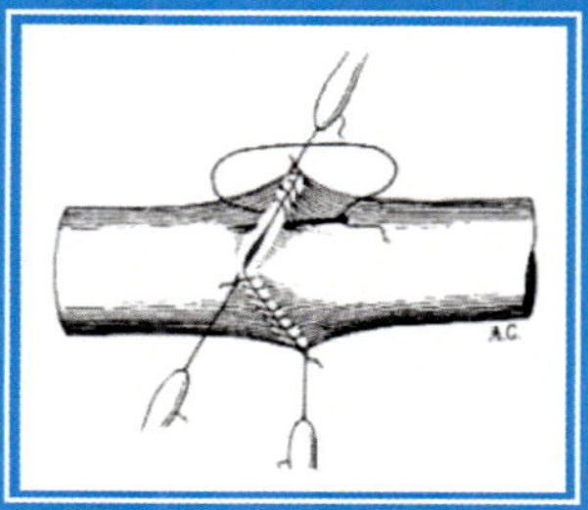

It is crucial each anastomosis performed during CABG be technically flawless and not have any kinks, pinched areas or wayward sutures. If the anastomosis is not correct, blood flow through the conduit will be impaired and the effectiveness of the operation vastly reduced, if not negated. The anastomosis also cannot have any gaps or it will leak, causing dangerous bleeding.

Another common conduit is a patient's vein, and the **Greater Saphenous Vein** (GSV) of the leg is usually used. Years ago, the process to harvest the GSV involved a long incision down the length of the leg, which patients from that era often report was more troublesome than the chest incision! A few surgeons still use the long-incision method, but most now use a method called **Endoscopic Vein Harvest** (**EVH**).

EVH uses a video camera and several small incisions to remove the vein. For my cases, a **Physician's Assistant (PA)** performs an ultrasound in the OR after the patient is asleep, in order to assess which leg has a higher-quality GSV (judging by its size and the thickness of the vein wall). The PA performs EVH while I harvest the LIMA. The length of vein harvested depends on the number of bypass grafts we are planning to do.

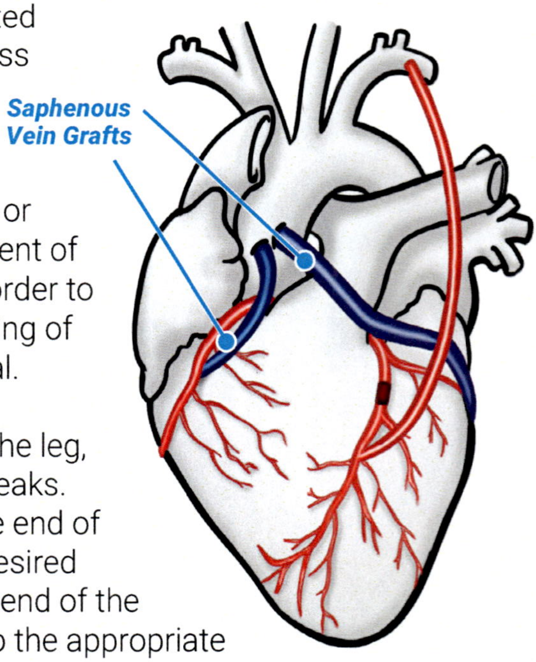

Once the GSV is ready to be
two ends of the vein are ligated, or
which had traveled in that segment of
way to the next-nearest vein in order to
Some patients experience swelling of
two but this goes back to normal.

Once the vein is removed from the leg,
are carefully tied off to prevent leaks.
ready to be used as conduit: one end of
connected to the **target** — the desired
coronary artery — and the other end of the
the aorta, after being trimmed to the appropriate length. This new pathway for blood to flow is called a saphenous vein graft, aka **SVG**.

Veins have valves in them, which allow blood to flow only in one direction toward the heart and not pool in the legs due to gravity. Care is taken during CABG to orient each vein graft in the opposite direction, so the valves do not hinder the blood flow.

If another bypass graft is needed, the process is repeated: sewing one end of another section of vein to the coronary target and the other end to the aorta, taking care to properly orient the vein. The process is repeated for as many bypass grafts as needed.

If you have varicose veins, please be sure to let your surgeon know, because your Greater Saphenous Vein may or may not be suitable for use. This is also true if you have had a bypass operation on your legs — your GSV may have already been used. If your veins are not usable, your surgeon will figure out a plan to work around this issue by using alternative conduits.

One alternative conduit is the **RIMA**. It is similar to the LIMA but located on the right side of the chest. It works very well as a conduit but is used in <10% of CABG cases nationwide. A lot of surgeons say they don't use it because the risk of chest wound problems is higher when the RIMA is used; plus, the operation takes longer.

However, the risk of wound problems only increases from about 1% to 2% and with efficient technique, the operation only takes about 15 minutes longer. Since it is such a good conduit, I use it about 80% of the time but not on very elderly or obese patients.

The **radial artery** is another option to use as conduit for CABG. The radial artery is one of the two arteries in the arm (ulnar is the other), extending from your elbow to your wrist, so blood flow to the hand is not messed up when the radial artery is taken out. Typically, the non-dominant arm is used; harvesting the radial artery does not weaken or harm the hand, however, and the artery can be taken from the dominant arm if needed.

The radial artery is particularly muscular and thick, and can easily spasm after surgery, reducing the blood flow. In fact, the spasm can be so strong that the bypass graft stops working.

Because of its propensity to spasm, many surgeons do not use the radial artery very much. I use it in certain circumstances, such as a young patient with blockages >90%, since very tight blockages seem to lessen spasm of the radial graft.

TAKE HOME POINTS

When it comes to CABG conduit:

The LIMA is pretty-much always used.

SVGs are usually used.

The RIMA is sometimes used — I myself use it a lot.

The radial artery is occasionally used.

Everything else is pretty-much never used.

MORE SURGICAL DETAILS...

A general anesthetic is used for CABG, which means you'll be completely asleep for the entire operation. You will have no awareness of the operation and no memory of it. The skeletal muscles in your body will be relaxed; you will be so relaxed, in fact, that you will not breathe on your own. So, a machine — a mechanical **ventilator** — will push air into the lungs to cause you to breathe.

A breathing tube is placed by the cardiac anesthesiologist once you have fallen asleep, to allow air to get into your lungs from the machine. A couple of special IVs will be placed as well to give you medications and allow specialized pressure monitoring of your heart.

At that time, a Foley catheter will be placed into the bladder by one of the OR nurses to monitor urine output. Antibiotics are given through your IV. The chest and legs are carefully cleansed. A "time-out" is performed allowing everyone in the room to confirm we have the correct patient and the correct operation.

The Cardiac Anesthesiologist performs a TEE, gently guiding the probe down the esophagus. As you know, the TEE provides ultrasound images of the heart as it moves. The TEE shows whether the heart muscle is strong or weak and provides information about how well the heart valves are opening and closing. If any unexpected issue of concern is seen, we discuss the issue as a team and determine if a change to the operative plan is needed.

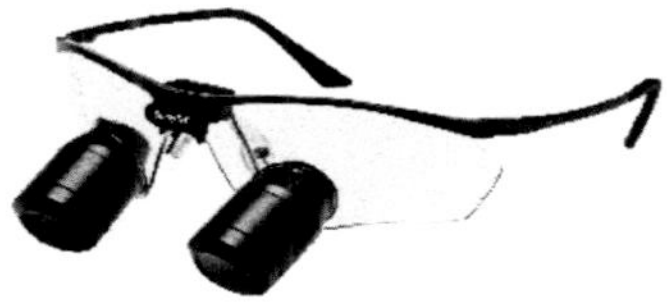

Like most heart surgeons, I put on special glasses called **loupes**, which magnify the structures of the heart. The coronary artery targets are small, usually around 1-2mm in size, which is roughly the thickness of a dime. My loupes are 3.5X, which make the coronaries appear 3 ½ times larger than normal.

I cleanse my hands with an alcohol-based cleanser, then don a sterile gown and gloves.

The operation begins! I carefully incise the skin with a scalpel. The incision is oriented up and down in the middle of the chest.

Patients often ask how long their incision will be: I tell them it will be just the right length. A cheesy answer, I admit, but the measured length of incision varies since the length of the breastbone varies person to person. Take a moment and feel your **sternal notch**, the bony V at the bottom of your neck. Then feel your **xiphoid** cartilage, the bumpy area at the top of your abdomen/bottom of your breast bone. I can usually start the incision a half-inch below the sternal notch and a half-inch above the xiphoid, keeping the incision as small as feasible.

The breastbone itself is cut with a surgical saw; this type of incision is called a **median sternotomy**.

I prepare, or harvest, the LIMA, separating it from the surrounding structures until it is free enough to reach the LAD without tension. I also harvest the RIMA if needed. My PA performs EVH to remove the needed length of vein from the leg.

Heparin, an anticoagulant, is given in a large dose, so blood does not clot inside the tubing of the heart-lung machine. Keeping track of how much heparin is given is crucial during heart bypass.

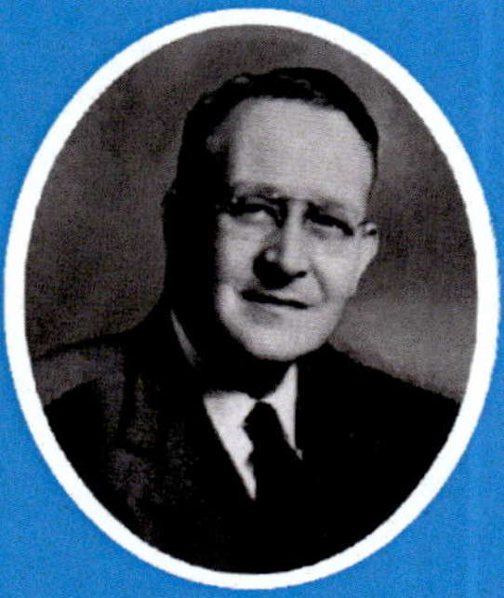

COULD YOU DO THAT?

Jay McLean discovered **heparin** in **1916**. By accident! He was studying extracts from the brain, trying to identify chemicals which *cause* clotting. He decided to study extracts from a **dog's liver** and identified a chemical which prevented clotting. He did this as a **second year medical student**! The chemical was named heparin by McLean's faculty adviser, using the Greek root for liver "**hepar**" — from which also comes hepatology, the study of the liver [87]. Currently, most heparin comes from **pig intestines** [88].

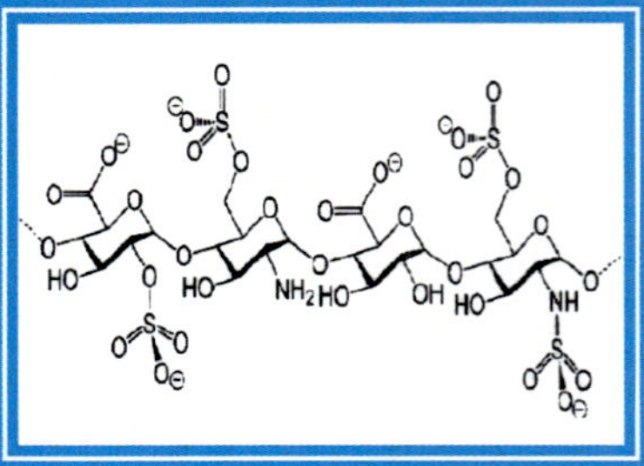

Heparin chemical structure

A small plastic tube called a **cannula** is placed into the aorta and another cannula placed in the right atrium; these are connected to the **heart-lung machine**. The heart-lung machine is also known as the "cardiopulmonary bypass (CPB) circuit." Most people find "heart-lung machine" easier to say! The machine pumps blood and moves air (oxygen and carbon dioxide), thereby functioning as the heart and lungs.

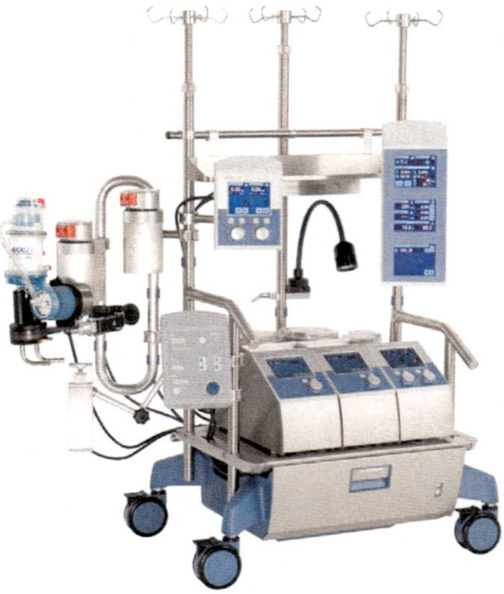

The heart-lung machine is started, pulling blood out of the right atrium, putting oxygen into it, and then returning it to the body via the aorta. A specialist called a **perfusionist** runs the heart-lung machine. Close communication between surgeon, perfusionist and cardiac anesthesiologist is paramount.

The heart is stopped by injecting a special chemical rich in potassium called **cardioplegia** into the coronary arteries; this chemical makes the myocardial cells unable to contract. Ice is put on the heart to cool it, in order to slow down cellular metabolism.

A clamp is placed on the aorta between the heart and the cannula in the aorta, so the warm blood returning from the heart-lung machine does not go backward into the heart and warm it up. The Cardiac Anesthesiologist turns the ventilator off, to keep the lungs from inflating and deflating and moving the heart around.

At this time, the EKG is flat, and there is no pulse. This situation can be off-putting for trainees! The EKG is flat because there is no electrical activity in the heart, and there is no pulse because the heart-lung machine moves the blood at a steady pressure. The heart is not moving at all, and it is smaller because it is empty, since all of the blood is taken out by the heart-lung machine. This is all amazing to see for the first time! Actually, it is pretty amazing every time I see it.

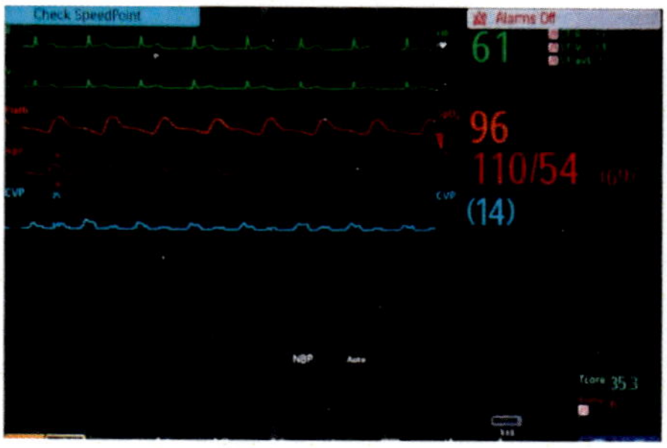

Normal EKG = heart beating

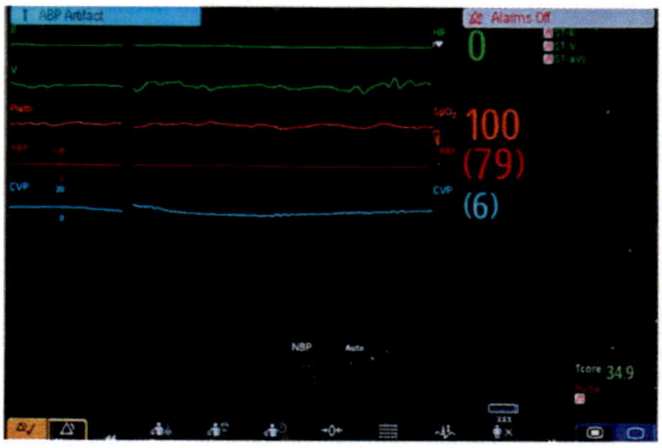

Flat EKG = heart stopped

Using current methods, the heart can be safely stopped for about 4 hours. After 4 hours, there can be significant damage to the myocardium and the heart may struggle to function once restarted. Most bypass operations are much shorter than this; still, we do not want to stop the heart for a second more than necessary. I often joke with my team members about someone wasting nano-seconds, as a way of expressing attention to the preciousness of time when the heart is stopped.

Typically in my operations, the heart is stopped for 30-45 minutes in order to complete 3 bypasses.

COULD YOU DO THAT?

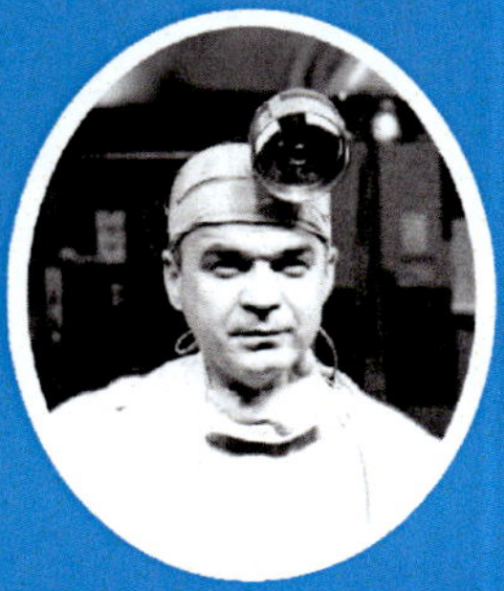

Dr. Walton Lillehei in Minnesota pioneered a method of heart surgery he called "**controlled cross circulation**." Used before the heart-lung machine was developed, his technique involved linking a child's circulation to a **parent**'s circulation. The parent's heart provided the force to move the child's blood during the operation. He was criticized for his operation having a **risk of 200% mortality**. He had good results but abandoned the technique after 45 operations, as the heart-lung machine technology became available and proved superior [89].

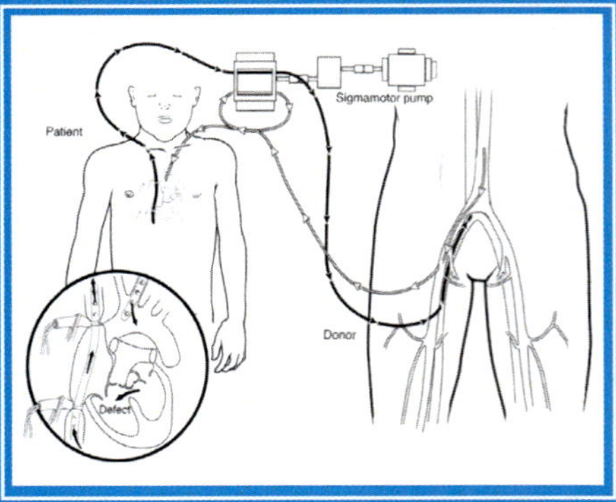

Once the heart is stopped, the bypass grafts are created. A coronary artery is identified and the location of the blockage identified. I usually prefer to start with the RCA in a 3-vessel CABG, but the order is not crucial. The sites of blockages are already known from the cardiac catheterization, and a location past the blockage is found — the **target**. The artery is opened with a tiny knife and the end of the vein sewn to the opening in the artery — this connection is the **distal anastomosis**. The other end of the vein is sewn to a small hole made in the aorta, just above the aortic valve, creating the **proximal anastomosis**.

This process is repeated for all of the bypass grafts needed, with the LIMA sewn to the LAD in almost all cases.

If any additional work needs to be done on the heart, such as repair or replacement of a valve, the heart is opened and the additional steps completed.

Once the bypass grafts and other work have been finished, the heart is restarted. To do this, warm water is poured on the heart and the potassium-based cardioplegia flushed out. The clamp on the aorta is removed.

Usually, the heart restarts on its own and it doesn't need an electrical shock; only every once in a while does it need a shock to get going. Some patients seem to worry their heart may not restart, but this is virtually unheard-of with modern techniques, and I have never had a heart fail to restart in thousands of operations.

In those uncommon cases when a shock is needed, nurses sometimes yell "CLEAR!" before delivering the electrical shock. I think they get this from TV or the movies, because the gloves worn by the surgical team insulate us from conduction of the electricity; we can safely touch the patient and the yelling is unnecessary. Of note, the paddles used to deliver a shock during heart surgery are small and can fit snuggly against the heart, unlike the bulky paddles used outside the body as seen on TV.

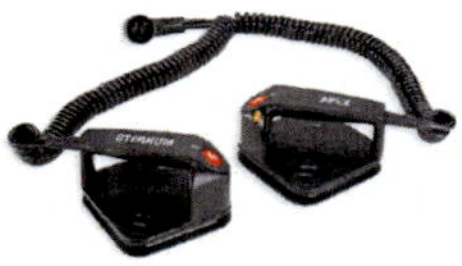

External Paddles

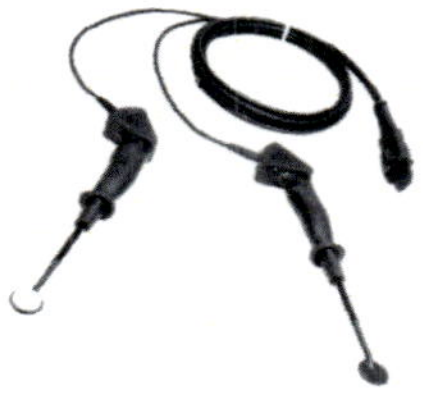

Internal Paddles

TAKE HOME POINTS

The heart-lung machine allows you to stay alive while your heart is stopped.

Take a peaceful rest & don't worry — your heart WILL restart.

Be sure to never roll your eyes at the nurse — this point is for surgeons!

Once the heart is beating, small electrical wires are placed known as temporary **pacing wires**: One end of each wire rests on the surface of the heart and the other end is brought through the skin and can be hooked to a temporary pacemaker. The wires allow the heart rate to be sped up if too slow in the ICU. The wires are removed in 1-2 days once the heart rate proves to be normal.

Chest tubes are also placed; I usually place 3 tubes. They are about the size of your pinky and quite long. One end of each tube sits within the chest and the other end is brought through the skin and attached to a collection chamber. The tubes help prevent accumulation of fluid and blood around the heart.

By the time the tubes are placed, the heart has been beating for several minutes and has regained most of its strength. The ventilator is restarted and the lungs are re-inflated. The heart-lung machine is slowly turned down so that the heart fills with blood and begins to pump the blood out. TEE is performed again, showing the heart muscle as it squeezes and the valves opening and closing.

Once we know the heart is pumping well with good strength, the heart-lung machine is turned off. The heart and lungs are back to doing all of the work to move the blood and exchange oxygen and carbon dioxide. At this point the myocardium is receiving more blood flow and more oxygen than when the operation began, since blood is flowing through the bypass grafts.

The cannulas in the aorta and right atrium are removed. A dose of **protamine** is given which counteracts heparin, so the blood will clot again.

EXTRA CREDIT

Protamine sulfate was initially derived from the sperm of salmon. Who figures this kind of stuff out?! Why would a chemical within salmon sperm counteract a chemical in dog liver?

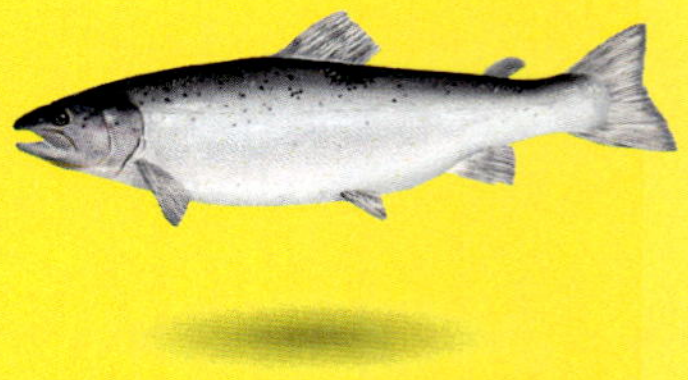

Protamine can cause allergic reactions in patients with allergies to fish and in men who have undergone vasectomy. Currently, protamine is typically made using recombinant technology (from DNA) [90].

Once the blood is clotting again, I carefully look at each structure in the chest to find any potential source of bleeding. Once I know nothing is bleeding, I close the chest wound.

Stainless steel wires are placed around the breastbone and tightened, pulling the edges of bone back together. Once the bone has healed weeks later, the wires are no longer needed, but there's usually no reason to take them out unless the patient has surgery again for some reason. The wires do not set off a metal detector – patients often ask about that. The wires are also safe for an MRI.

Dissolvable sutures are placed under the skin to close the wound, and the top layer of skin is sealed with medical-grade glue. Dressings are placed.

And that's it! The operation is over.

A three-vessel CABG usually takes me and my team about **3-4 hours** skin-to-skin, meaning from the first incision to the last dab of glue. Efficiency is desirable, since we don't want an operation to last any longer than it has to. Still, my mindset is to spend whatever time it takes to do each step properly and in the correct order. I am committed to staying as long as it takes to provide an outstanding operation.

TAKE HOME POINTS

Heart bypass surgery involves hundreds of steps.

Despite the complexity, a flawless operation is possible when every step is performed correctly & in the correct order.

"Triple bypass" is how a layperson often describes a three-vessel bypass. I prefer to say "CABBAGE times 3," written **CABG x3**. The most common heart bypass surgery performed in the USA is CABG x3.

NUMBER OF BYPASSES		
1	**"Single"**	**CABG x 1**
2	**"Double"**	**CABG x 2**
3	**"Triple"**	**CABG x 3**
4	**"Quadruple"**	**CABG x 4**
5	**"Quintuple"**	**CABG x 5**

I have occasionally performed 6 bypass grafts but not more than that; it is rare for there to be that many coronary arteries or branches large enough to graft.

A general objective of CABG is **complete revascularization**, the idea of providing a bypass graft to any and all major arteries and large branches which have a severe blockage. It basically means our objective is to fix every artery that needs it and no arteries with blockages should be left without improved blood flow.

TAKE HOME POINTS

Complete revascularization ==>
if we are going in there at all,
we're gonna fix everything that needs to be fixed.

RISKS

Welcome to a section most patients would be happy to skip over. Who wants to read about all the bad things that can happen? Pretty much nobody. I understand. I am an optimist, and I do not spend a lot of time thinking about negative possibilities. I only have the mental capacity to worry about actual problems, not theoretical ones! However, it is important for you to know the risks associated with CABG, so that you can make an informed decision about undergoing the surgery.

Fortunately, heart bypass surgery is safer now than in years past, certainly safer than 30, 20 or even 10 years ago. It is safer because CABG is one of the most studied operations in existence, and we heart surgeons are constantly working to improve the operation. Heart surgeons collectively have labored for decades to understand the best way to care for patients who need heart surgery.

Part of the improvement in safety has been the rise of **team** culture. Whereas decades ago, a surgeon might think he (or she) was more important than everyone else and acted like it, now most surgeons are attuned to the value of the team. The surgeon trope of conceited superiority can still be seen lingering via movies and television – ala Dr. Strange in the Marvel Cinematic Universe, a neurosurgeon it is worth noting! – but not so much in real life.

Surgeons are trained to depend on their own abilities. Well, not just surgeons – pretty much all of us. This self-reliance begins early in life in Western society. Who can recall taking a group test in high school? Not me. Might've been nice. I made it through grade school, middle school, high school, college and medical school taking tests by myself. And then all of a sudden when I became a surgeon, I'm supposed to work well with others?! Go figure.

DO YOU KNOW?

How many tests does one have to pass to become a heart surgeon?
2,500!

Well, ok, I made that answer up.
But the path to becoming a heart surgeon is a long and often lonely one.

The path classically has involved:
4 years of medical school
then 5 years of General Surgery residency
then 2-3 years of Cardiac Surgery fellowship.

No wonder surgeons tend to be grumpy, given all that testing & training!

But as I have gained experience as a surgeon, I have come to better understand and appreciate the team I lead. I realize that *my* success is not my success at all, it is *our* success as a team. There is no way I can pull off a heart bypass operation by myself. For instance, I don't know how to administer an anesthetic. I don't know how to run the heart-lung machine. I don't know how to assist myself. I don't know the official names of all the instruments (I made up my own names for many of them). I don't know where supplies are stored in the OR area.

Hmmm... it occurs to me that I don't know a lot! But the cardiac anesthesiologist, the perfusionist, the PA, the **scrub tech** and the **circulator nurse** know these things. Our collective knowledge and expertise is impressive.

TAKE HOME POINTS

I know a thing or two about heart surgery.

The TEAM knows more.

Each person is crucial to the operation; that is, the operation cannot happen without each team member. It is impossible for one person to perform heart surgery.

When the team is working well, our work is a beautiful thing. It resembles a well-choreographed dance by an expert troupe, where each move is in sync, on time, in place. It also like an elite SWAT or SEAL team, where each member is depending on another, so that everyone stays safe and the mission accomplished.

Beyond the OR team, a larger team is crucial to your care. The cardiologist makes the diagnosis of CAD and guides your overall care, including your medications. My office assistant coordinates logistical arrangements with the hospital. Nurse Practitioners help care for you before and after surgery. Internal Medicine doctors manage medical problems before and after surgery. The nurses care for you, and Respiratory Therapists and Physical Therapists coach you on breathing and walking. The list goes on. The team is large and every person is important.

I feel like the quarterback of a winning football team. I lead the plays and get credit for the wins. But no quarterback wins as a one-man team. Tom Brady would not win a football game playing by himself against a high school team. Because no one person can perform every task in a complex system. In the same way, the best surgeon on earth cannot get you through heart surgery alone.

I know this. I know the team around me is what is successful. I am blessed to be surrounded by outstanding people, professionals dedicated to helping you. With outstanding people, we — your team — are able to provide outstanding care.

When it comes to risk, the team and the care we provide are only as strong as the weakest link. I am obsessed with surgical technique, with technical perfection — making every cut and putting every stitch exactly where it needs to be — and I do not make many errors in technique. I have trained my mind to anticipate errors even before they occur, to know when they are *likely* to occur. I tell my kids I treat all of life like it's a trick question.

But no matter how careful I am, I make errors. Every human on earth makes errors; in fact, an unassisted human will make errors about 1% of the time [91]. When I make an error, I rely on my team members to catch it. And I catch theirs.

Of course, there are many more steps on your journey than just the operation itself, so striving for technical perfection in the OR is not enough. My team and I are committed to working toward perfection at every step. We may not *reach* perfection every time, but we are aiming for it. Every one of us wants to see you do extremely well.

While expecting you to do well, I need you to know there are risks to every surgery. I will discuss with you the particular risks you face based on your particular anatomy, medical problems, and circumstance.

That being said, in general, most patients who come from home and have a scheduled CABG on a strong heart have a risk of dying of roughly 1%. I recommend dwelling on the 99% chance of living! The risk may be higher if you are old — oh, sorry, I meant "advanced in age" — or had a heart attack or if the heart is weak or for a number of reasons, which is why it is important to discuss your particular risks.

For all patients, there are also risks of bleeding, stroke, and wound problems, as well as kidney dysfunction. There are other complications which happen only rarely, such as a need for a permanent pacemaker or bypass grafts which do not work correctly, or even a heart attack.

Another risk is that the bypasses do not last long. **Patency** is the term used to describe whether the bypass grafts are working, that is, whether they are open or not. When a graft is open and blood is moving through it, the graft is patent. The patency of the LIMA to LAD graft has been extensively studied and can be expected to be 95% at 15 years; this means the LIMA graft has a 95% chance of still being open and working in 15 years. Thank you, LIMA endothelium and your splendid nitric oxide!

The patency of vein grafts is lower, around 50% at 10 years. If a bypass graft loses patency and becomes blocked or completely closed, it may cause angina or even a heart attack, or it may not affect the heart in a measurable way — it all depends on the particular circumstance.

TAKE HOME POINTS

For most patients, the risk of death from CABG is low & the patency of bypass grafts is high for many years.

If a graft loses patency, the treatment varies: some patients may need a stent while some patients may need to undergo CABG again; sometimes nothing needs to be done. Redo CABG is usually reserved for cases where several or all of the bypass grafts have lost patency, which is usually many years after the first bypass surgery.

Another risk of CABG is **atrial fibrillation**, which is often shortened to "Afib." Afib is an irregular heart rhythm, described as "irregularly irregular" as some sort of medical establishment inside joke. Around 30% of patients who undergo CABG develop afib after the operation, so a lot of patients deal with afib after surgery. Afib most commonly arises on Post-Op Day 2 or 3 [92].

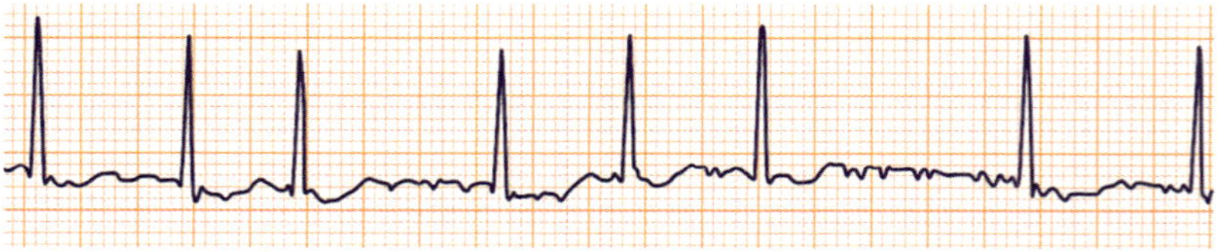

Atrial fibrillation on EKG

Afib can make you feel more tired than you otherwise would, since blood moves a bit less efficiently when your heart rhythm is haphazard. Some patients can feel the irregularity of the heart beat itself, as if it is pounding – this sensation is called **palpitations**. Some patients do not sense when they are in afib.

Afib does not usually degenerate into a "worse" rhythm; however, the heart rate can be high, sometimes over 150 beats per minute, a condition known as Rapid Ventricular Response (**RVR**). With the heart rate so high and slightly erratic, the blood pressure can drop. These effects can make a patient feel dizzy or unsteady.

The biggest danger with afib is formation of a blood clot (thrombus). Because blood does not move as efficiently through the heart, it can stagnate in certain areas, particularly in an outpouching of the left atrium called the **left atrial appendage**. Stagnating blood will tend to clot, and it is thought that up to 90% of blood clots which form due to afib occur in the left atrial appendage. If a blood clot forms there or anywhere in the heart, it can move out and go to the brain, causing a stroke.

To prevent this, most patients with afib are treated with an anti-coagulant to help prevent a blood clot from forming.

EXTRA CREDIT

Anti-coagulants are called "blood thinners" by almost everyone, including healthcare professionals.

However, this is a misnomer because anti-coagulants do not affect the viscosity of the blood in any appreciable way; that is, they do not change the thinness or thickness of the blood. [93]

The anti-coagulant classically used to treat afib is **coumadin**. There are also newer agents such as Eliquis and Xarelto, which are more convenient for patients because they do not require blood tests.

Needless to say, we want to avoid afib; unfortunately, no method of preventing afib after heart surgery has been found. We try to reduce the number of patients who get it, but afib still happens to some patients. Older patients tend to be particularly susceptible to getting afib.

Fortunately, most patients who develop afib after CABG will find relief; in fact, up to 90% of patients will not have afib 3 months after operation [94], so it tends to be a short-term issue after CABG. We can often hasten its resolution with medications, such as a beta-blocker or **amiodarone**.

We can also perform **cardioversion**, which shocks the heart back into a normal rhythm. Oftentimes we do not perform cardioversion soon after operation because the afib is fairly likely to come back until the inflammation within the chest heals. Long term, if all else fails and afib does not resolve, an **ablation** can be done to help restore a normal rhythm.

TAKE HOME POINTS

Afib

Is an irregular heart rhythm common after CABG.

Usually resolves within 3 months after CABG.

Is treated with beta-blockers & amiodarone.

Typically requires anti-coagulation until it goes away & stays away.

OFF-PUMP BYPASS

It is possible to do bypass surgery without the heart-lung machine; this method is called **Off-Pump** (**OPCAB**), because the pump of the heart-lung machine is not used. In conversations about CABG, if the On- or Off-pump designation is not mentioned, then it is assumed the pump/heart-lung machine is used.

There are some potential advantages in not using the heart-lung machine. The amount of inflammation is less, since blood does not contact the plastic of the machine's tubing. There may be a slightly lower risk of stroke, as well as kidney malfunction. The need for blood transfusion is also less.

But scientific studies have not shown these advantages to be as reliable as one might think. There have been a few studies showing superiority of Off-Pump CABG over On-Pump, but there are even more studies showing no difference or showing superiority of On-Pump bypass. One drawback with Off-Pump CABG — and likely why the data does not consistently show Off-Pump to be better — is that with the heart still moving, connecting the small blood vessels is difficult. It is easier for the anastomosis to get messed up, which vastly reduces the benefit of the operation and may cause complications.

Since the data is all over the place, it is not clear which method is better, although it is important to know patients do well with both methods; it is more a question of which method is *best* for a given patient. Many surgeons such as myself have interpreted the overall findings to mean that the best method of bypass operation is the one the surgeon is most adept at performing. If a surgeon is great at Off-Pump, then that is the best operation to have with that surgeon. If a surgeon is great at On-Pump, then On-Pump is the best to have with that surgeon.

Roughly 80-85% of CABGs in the USA involve the heart-lung machine and 15-20% of CABGs are Off-Pump [95]. Most surgeons prefer to use the heart-lung machine.

TAKE HOME POINTS

Off-pump & On-pump CABG are both excellent options for most patients.

I do not usually perform CABG Off-Pump unless I have a specific reason to do so, meaning there is an unusual circumstance for which I think Off-pump is the best option for a particular patient. In my experience, having the heart completely motionless while creating the anastomoses, by using the On-Pump technique, affords the highest quality operation and the best outcome for most of my patients.

CAN'T WE DO IT SOME OTHER WAY?

Most CABGs are performed with median sternotomy and the heart-lung machine. Still, a lot of patients ask about alternatives: Can a small incision be used? Can you avoid "cracking" my chest?
The answer is, Sometimes.

MID-CAB is a minimally-invasive method of performing bypass using the LIMA to the LAD. MID-CAB is short for **M**inimally **I**nvasive **D**irect **C**oronary **A**rtery **B**ypass, pronounced "Mid-Cab." For some reason, no one says "Mid-CABG." It involves no cutting of the breastbone.
A roughly 1 ½ inch incision is made on the left side of the chest, not far from the nipple. The incision is oriented left and right instead of up and down like a median sternotomy.

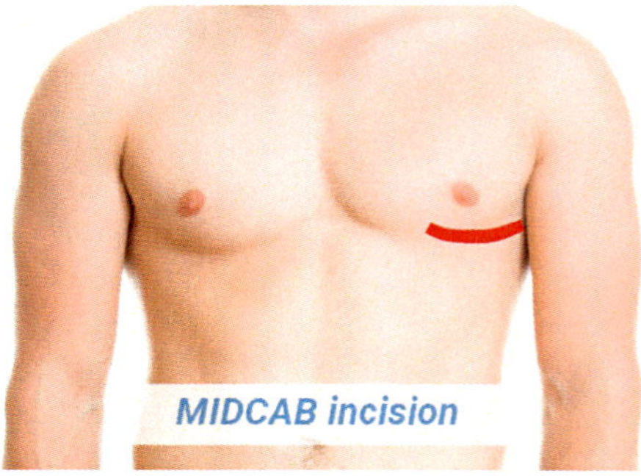

The LIMA is harvested through this incision and an anastomosis performed connecting the LIMA to LAD. This is usually performed Off-Pump, because it is difficult to stop the heart using this approach. It is not usually feasible to perform multiple bypasses with this method since access to the heart is limited. The operation takes 2-3 hours to perform.

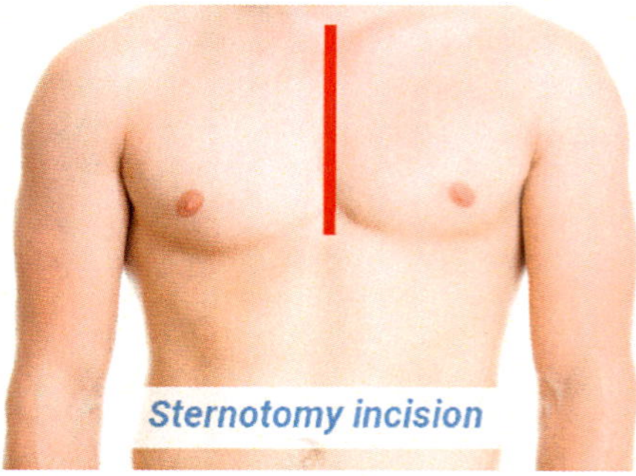

Nation-wide, MID-CAB operations are not performed very often: It is rare for a patient to only need one bypass graft; indeed, only about 3-4% of CABG patients undergo LIMA to LAD and nothing else. So the majority of patients having CABG would not achieve complete revascularization with MID-CAB by itself.

To provide an option for patients with multi-vessel CAD, some surgeons promote a hybrid approach, combining CABG and PCI. The hybrid approach uses a LIMA to LAD via MID-CAB, combined with coronary stents to address other blockages.

The coronary stents are placed by an interventional cardiologist, typically a few days after MID-CAB, which is a day or two before the patient goes home. Sometimes the care team decides to wait a couple of weeks before placing the stents. A hybrid approach has not been popular at my hospital, and our team does not use the method regularly, though it can be a good option for some patients.

The potential benefits of MID-CAB are avoidance of sternotomy, less blood transfusion, and slightly lower risk of stroke. However, the drawback is limited visibility and the difficulty of creating the anastomosis through a small incision with the heart moving. Plus, the ribs are spread to allow access to the anatomy, which causes pain. Finally, it is difficult to do any bypass grafts other than the LIMA to LAD.

Due to these limitations, I do not perform MID-CAB with any regularity; instead, the minimally-invasive option I offer is Robotic CABG.

Robotic CABG involves use of the Da Vinci surgical robot, a system developed by Intuitive Surgical. Since it is difficult to sew using small suture with the robot, most surgeons such as myself use the robot to harvest the LIMA and then sew the anastomosis to the LAD by hand through one of the incisions. Purists call this Robotic-Assisted CABG.

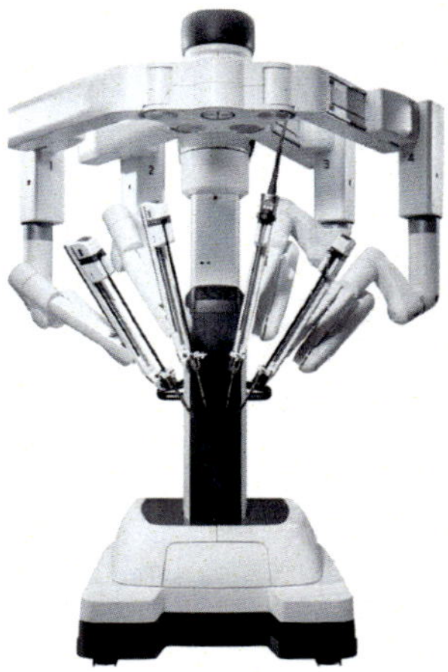

DaVinci Robot

Keep in mind that the "robot" does not know how to do anything; that is, it does not make any movements on its own. The surgeon does not push START and go play golf; I'm sure

Cyberdyne — oops, I meant Intuitive Surgical — is working on that. But for now the robot cannot do anything on its own, go rogue or become "self-aware."

The term robot, then, is a bit of a misnomer; rather, the device is a form of **telesurgery** where the movements of the surgeon at the controls are translated into movements of the instruments, allowing for small incisions and high precision.

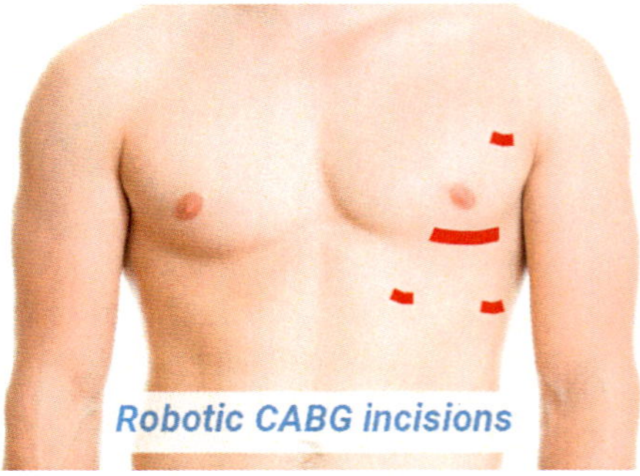
Robotic CABG incisions

The breastbone is not cut with Robotic CABG. Four small incisions are made in the left chest, each about ½ inch in size. A video camera and two robot instruments are placed through the small incisions. The LIMA is harvested using these tools. Once the LIMA is fully prepared, the robot is removed and the LIMA to LAD anastomosis is performed Off-Pump through one of the incisions, which is enlarged slightly.

The benefits and drawbacks of Robotic CABG are similar to MID-CAB, though the incisions are smaller and thus there may be less pain. The video camera has 10X magnification — making the anatomy appear nearly 3 times as large as my loupes — so the visualization is superb.

While structures appear larger, the LAD can be difficult to identify with the robot, especially if the surface of the heart has a lot of fat on it. So when reviewing the cardiac cath prior to surgery, I usually like to see a plump distal LAD, which I know can be localized with the robot. If the LAD is small on cath, then I do not recommend Robotic CABG. Overall, I approach each patient with the intent to personalize the plan to his or her specific needs and anatomy to thereby determine the best method for revascularization. If a robotic approach fits the patient's needs, then it can be a great option.

TAKE HOME POINTS

Robotic CABG may be a good option for some patients.

WHAT TO EXPECT

"It's 90% mental. The other half is physical."
Yogi Berra [96]

BEFORE THE OPERATION

I believe it is important to plan and prepare well for bypass surgery, as most problems are best solved by prevention.

My office assistant will coordinate with you regarding logistics for your operation, letting you know the date and time and where to go. If you are on Plavix or an anti-coagulant such as coumadin, it needs to be stopped prior to operation; my assistant will let you know exactly when — usually at least 7 days ahead. A baby Aspirin can be continued up to the night before surgery.

If you are coming from home for surgery, we ask you to come by the hospital one or two days prior to operation for **Pre-Admission Testing** (**PAT**).

Pre-Admission Testing generally includes:

Basics labs: To be sure you are not anemic or showing evidence of kidney problems.

COVID-19: Likely needed to allow admission to the hospital; the policies are frequently changing!

Type & Cross: To determine your blood type and prepare several units of blood in case they are needed during the operation. About 30% of patients undergoing bypass surgery require a blood transfusion sometime during their stay in the hospital. The blood is carefully screened and the risk of getting a communicable disease from blood is extremely low (roughly 1 in 250,000).

If your religious beliefs include a conviction that blood transfusion is not acceptable (i.e., Jehovah's Witness), let me know so we can discuss plans for your particular case.

Family members often ask about donating blood for their loved one but this is not feasible.

5 meter walk test: We ask you to walk 5 meters (roughly 15 feet) and a staff member will determine how long it takes. You can use a cane or walker if you usually do.

Patients who can walk 5m in less than 7 seconds are generally fit enough to undergo bypass surgery. If it takes longer than 7 seconds then we will need to discuss the results and may need to consider alternative options to surgery, since you may have too tough a time getting around after operation.

PFTs: Pulmonary Function Tests — to measure your lung capacity. If lung function is poor, we will need to discuss the results: sometimes CABG can still be performed safely and sometimes not. Often the lung function is poor for patients who have smoked cigarettes for many years, indicative of COPD.

Carotid duplex ultrasound: An ultrasound of the carotid arteries in the neck. Patients with CAD can have blockages in the carotid arteries, and if a severe blockage is found, we will need to address it. In most cases we perform CABG first and then clean out the carotid plaque (a procedure called carotid endarterectomy) 3-4 months later.

CXR - Chest x-ray: To assess the size and position of the heart and lungs.

Some of the paperwork related to your admission can be done at PAT: i.e., signatures ad infinitum. Meanwhile, my office assistant will contact your insurance company for pre-approval for surgery, when applicable.

An Internal Medicine doctor may meet with you during your Pre-Admission Testing and help take care of you after surgery. We certainly don't want any of your medical problems to be neglected!

The night before surgery, do not eat or drink any food or water after midnight. In some cases, you can take medications after midnight with a sip of water, if advised by me or the anesthesiologist to do so.

I would recommend packing a small bag for the hospital, but there is no need to bring luggage. You may want to bring your favorite toothpaste and deodorant, as well as a book to read. Please leave valuables at home, including cash and jewelry. Your wedding ring will need to be removed for surgery, so go ahead and leave it at home. Many patients bring a cell phone with them, which is fine, but it is probably best to assume anything you bring with you will be lost.

Try to get to sleep at a reasonable hour, as we will be expecting you at the hospital early. Admittedly, a number of patients have difficulty sleeping on the night before surgery.

As you go to sleep, I recommend reflecting on the blessings in your life. Then, allow your mind to envision your success at the end of your surgical journey. Create a scene in your mind: perhaps a splendid moment on vacation with your family or friends, celebrating your recovery. Or a successful meeting at work. Maybe a quiet walk with someone you love. Be as detailed as you can, in your mind. Then, perhaps you can pray and thank God for this vision. And for the strength you have now, the strength you will have then, and the good you will do with the strength you receive.

TAKE HOME POINTS

Be thankful for your blessings.

Expect to do amazingly well. Then you will!

DAY OF SURGERY

Time to wake up early! My office assistant will let you know what time to arrive but it is commonly 5:30 am for surgery at 7:15 am.

Come into the hospital Main Entrance and check in at the front desk. A staff member will direct you to the Pre-Op area.

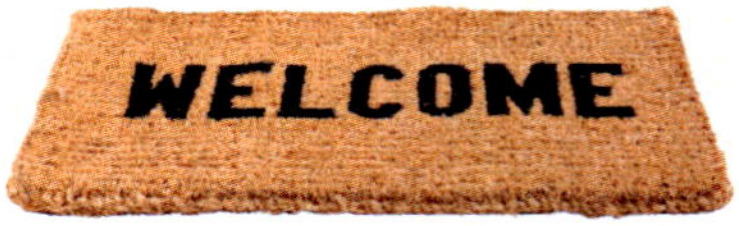

In Pre-Op, you'll be provided a hospital gown to put on. A technician will come and shave your chest and legs, if needed.

I usually stop by the Pre-Op area around 7:00 am. I am happy to discuss any last-minute questions or concerns you may have. I also typically offer to pray with my patients if that is something you would appreciate. You will meet your cardiac anesthesiologist in Pre-Op as well; feel free to ask him or her any questions about going to sleep or special concerns you may have, such as what to do about dentures or hearing aids.

You will meet the OR circulator nurse, who will confirm your identity and look over the consent forms to be sure they are in order.

Feel free to use the restroom in the Pre-Op area. But do not worry too much about getting your bladder empty because a Foley (bladder) catheter will be placed once you are asleep in the OR.

Once you are comfortable to proceed and the OR is ready, you will be wheeled into the OR on the hospital bed.

If you have friends or family with you, they are welcome to wait in the family waiting room. An OR staff member will plan to update them every hour or so, and I will plan to talk to them when the operation is complete.

In the OR, the circulator nurse will help you move over to the OR table; the table is narrow, so take your time. If there is some music you would like to hear, let the nurse know. The temperature in the OR is usually pretty low, and the nurse will be happy to get a blanket for you.

The anesthesiologist will place a fancy IV and give you a medication through the IV to help you drift off to sleep.

Next thing you know, you'll be waking up in the ICU and the operation will be completely over!

Some patients worry about waking up during the surgery. This is extremely rare with modern techniques. As a testament to the outstanding skill of the cardiac anesthesiologists with whom I work, I have never had a patient awaken during surgery in thousands of operations.

TAKE HOME POINTS

Expect to have an early morning & a great day.

IN THE ICU

As you wake in the ICU, you will have several tubes and fancy IVs. The experience of waking varies between patients, and it is hard to predict exactly what you will perceive and how you will feel. Some people wake up mellow and some people freak out big-time. Hopefully, you will be one of the mellow ones!

Most of the time, the breathing tube is still in place when the patient begins to awaken. I know a lot of patients are very worried about this ahead of time. It can be off-putting to wake up with the tube but most patients report to me later that it is not as bad as you would think. Many patients do not remember having the tube at all, even if they begin to awaken with the tube still in place.

We will get the tube out as soon as we safely can, as soon as you begin to breathe without much help from the ventilator. This is usually 2-4 hours after the end of the operation. Only in unusual situations is the tube kept in for longer.

We often put mittens on the patient's hands to prevent pulling at the tubes. I know this can be quite annoying to patients, once they realize mittens are there. If you are calm, the ICU nurse will usually be able to take the mittens off. A lot of patients are ready to have the breathing tube removed before they are conscious enough to be bothered by the mittens.

TAKE HOME POINTS

Don't worry about waking up with the breathing tube. It's easy!

Just open your eyes, stay mellow & we'll get it out as soon as we safely can.

After the breathing tube is removed, the ICU nurse will continue helping you with anything you need. You will need medicine for pain relief, and I usually order three or four different ones. Do not be shy asking for pain medicine. You may be quite sore the first night, and we will work to find a recipe of pain medicine effective to control the discomfort.

The ICU nurse will help you get out of bed to a chair. This is a process! It may take a while to get out of bed. Don't fret: Keep in mind you have many tubes and IVs plus your soreness slowing you down. Getting up will get easier each time.

You can start to eat and drink. Start slow, try some ice first. Then water. Then juice. Then a light meal. A lot of patients do not have much of an appetite for several days. You can have coffee, though I'd recommend going easy on caffeine and do not drink the coffee hot; ideally, you should probably wait a day or two on coffee unless it is decaffeinated.

Also, carbonated beverages are not ideal early on, since the carbon dioxide can distend your stomach and bowels, which are slowed by the anesthetic and pain meds. On the other hand, some patients find a bit of ginger ale can help soothe nausea and an upset stomach.

You will see a number of healthcare providers in the ICU, so do not be alarmed by all the attention.

A **Respiratory Therapist** will coach you on your breathing.

A **Physical Therapist** will help you take a walk.

A team of ICU doctors called Intensivists will help oversee your medical care while in the ICU.

You are likely to feel tired and sleep more than usual after the operation. This is expected and normal.

A family member is welcome to visit you in the ICU, which is not generally locked or restricted. Family members may be asked to step out of the room periodically in order to allow for certain aspects of care to be provided.

Also, night-time nurses seem to be a bit more sensitive to the presence of visitors, so please be open to their guidance on a good time to visit. Family members should not plan to stay all night in the ICU; there is nowhere for them to sleep, and you will NOT feel like sharing space in the bed!

TAKE HOME POINTS

You will be popular in the ICU!

POD 1

Assuming all goes as planned, you will be ready to leave the ICU the day after surgery, which we call Post-Op Day 1.

One or more of your chest tubes will be removed, depending on how much fluid is draining. This may take your breath away for a few seconds but is not generally painful. Overall the pain gets better for most patients after tubes come out, since the tubes tend to rub up against the ribs causing irritation.

The Foley (bladder) catheter is usually removed at this point as well. A couple of the special IVs placed in the OR can be removed.

Usually by lunch-time, most of the tubes and lines have been removed – you still have the temporary pacing wires, one or two chest tubes, and an IV. You will also notice several small pads taped to your chest, which provide a constant monitor of your heart rhythm.

You will likely be getting extra oxygen through a **nasal cannula**, a small tube that sits just below your nose. You will need this less and less as your breathing improves. The Respiratory Therapist and your nurse will let you know when you need to wear the extra oxygen. If the extra oxygen dries out your nasal passages, let the RT know so a humidifier can be added. Don't fret about the extra oxygen – almost all patients go home without extra oxygen unless they were using it prior to surgery.

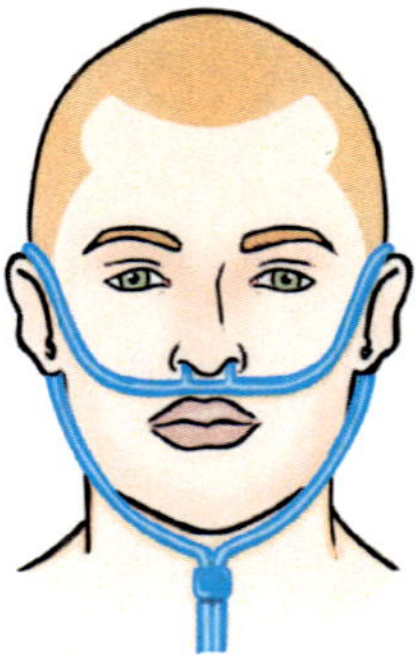

Time to walk! The ICU nurse or Physical Therapist will help with your first excursion. It may be short, only a few steps – just see what you can do. Like getting up to the chair, don't fret if your first walk is difficult. It will quickly become much easier.

Your new room will be on **Telemetry**, an area of the hospital where your heart rhythm is constantly monitored. Some people call it StepDown. The Telemetry nurse will take good care of you. If not, let me know! (We will move that nurse to the neurosurgery ward!) Our nurses are excellent, available and eager to help as needed – just push the button on the bedside remote.

In general, the Telemetry nurse will be in the room less often than the ICU nurse, since he or she covers more patients on Telemetry. Still, my team is committed to providing the care you need when you need it, so never be shy to let someone know what you need.

A family member can be with you in your room almost all the time on Telemetry. It is possible for a family member to stay in the room overnight. Sleep may prove hard to get, however!

Sleep can be elusive the first few nights: the pain and soreness, the beeping of monitors and alarms, the general bustle of the hospital.

The hospital bed, though it adjusts in multiple ways, often stirs up back pain. Staff members will be coming in to get labs and an x-ray almost every morning.

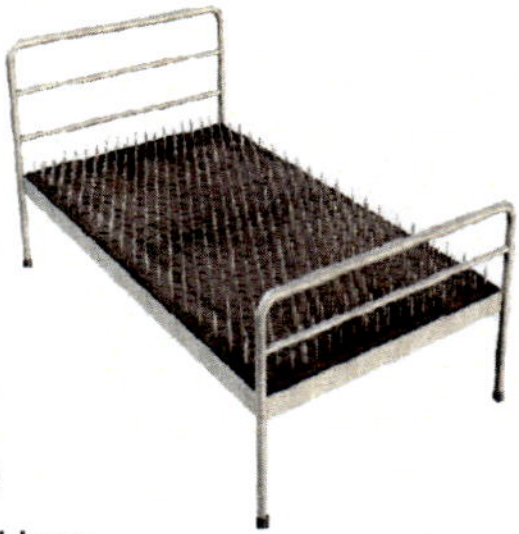

On top of these issues, a lot of patients have trouble laying flat at first and find sleeping in a recliner is better — please try that if you like. I don't tend to prescribe a "sleeping pill" but am usually willing to order one if you feel you need it. Your sleep will naturally improve as you heal and feel better and get back home to your own bed. Due to poor sleep at night, a lot of patients tell me they never took naps before but find themselves dozing off during the day while they recover. This is expected.

TAKE HOME POINTS

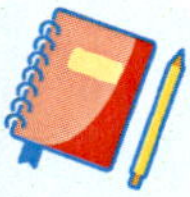

Get sleep whenever & however you can.

POD 2

Today, another chest tube will come out. Assuming your heart rhythm has been stable, your temporary pacing wires can be removed. Like the chest tubes, this may take your breath away but doesn't usually hurt.

You should plan to walk three times today: morning, afternoon, evening.

At this point, please get some help when you walk. If you need to get up to the restroom, get some help from a family member, Telemetry nurse or Physical Therapist. We definitely don't want you to trip and fall. As your strength and balance improve, you'll be able to get up and walk by yourself again.

You need to work on your breathing often. The Respiratory Therapist will teach you deep breathing exercises. You will be given a **PEP**, a plastic

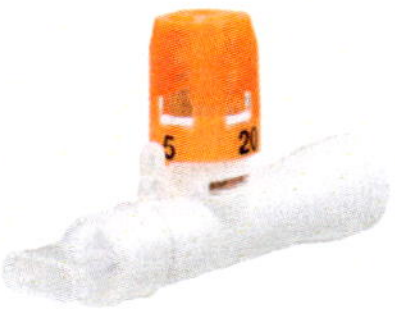

PEP

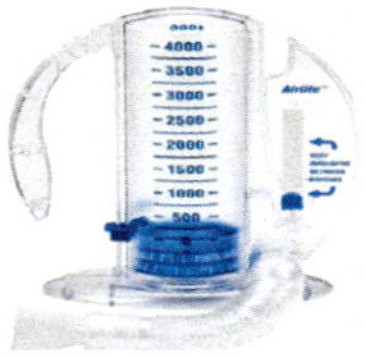

IS

device that helps strengthen your breathing — please use this every hour. You may also have an **incentive spirometer** (**IS**), which has a gauge to follow your progress.

Most patients rely on pain pills at this point, though the more powerful IV pain medicines are still available if you need them. It is important to take pain medicine consistently. Only you know how much pain and discomfort you are having, but I usually recommend some pain medicine every 4 hours, even if only Tylenol or Ibuprofen. This consistent dosing prevents the pain from getting out of control.

A lot of patients seem worried about getting addicted to pain medicines and decline to take pain pills. While addiction is a legitimate concern, it is highly unlikely you will become addicted to pain medicine when taking it appropriately after heart surgery. You have acute pain — that is, your pain started with the operation and will end when you heal — and you can expect to only need pain medicine for 1-2 weeks. Patients with chronic pain tend to have a much higher risk of addiction, since they get accustomed to pain medicine over many weeks or months and then cannot give it up. So, for a few days, get the pain medicine you need. Soon, you will not need any at all.

Some patients seem to want to prove how macho they are or how they can achieve mind over matter, so they avoid pain medicine and try to suffer through the pain. Men seem to be more stubborn than women in this regard.

LETS GET PERSONAL

When I was a boy, my grandfather was shot in the abdomen trying to stop a bank robbery. He underwent emergency surgery and survived, thank God. He thought he would heal quicker if he had no pain medicine, so he refused to take any. He was a macho man, to be sure, but his method was misguided and actually slowed his recovery.

We know from a medical point of view that you will recover faster if your pain is well-controlled rather than trying to suffer through it. If you try to simply grin and bear it, you will not be able to get out of bed, walk, and breathe deeply or perform the breathing exercises — all of the things that will enable you to get stronger and get home.

TAKE HOME POINTS

Don't be macho or stubborn — Be savvy!

Get the pain medicines you need.

You won't need any for long.

POD 3

You are getting close to going home!

Your last tube will be removed if still in place. You are getting up more, perhaps getting to the restroom by yourself. At night, I still recommend getting help so you do not fall, since the room is dark and unfamiliar.

You can take a shower. It is really more of a glorified spongebath but most patients feel refreshed afterward. It's interesting how the little things in life can matter so much when you haven't had them for a time! Definitely get a Telemetry nurse to help, so that you don't have trouble with your wound dressing or IV or heart monitor.

You may be nearly ready to have a bowel movement (a **BM** = going #2). Almost all patients experience slowing of the bowels during their recovery, and it is usually 3-4 days after surgery before a BM happens. You will be on a stool softener, and we can increase the amount of help even beyond that, all the way up to an enema.

But beware what you ask for! Sometimes the pendulum swings all the way over, if you know what I mean. Unless you are feeling distended and having pain, most of the time the bowels will wake up just fine and not much "help" is needed. When you do get a chance to reign on the porcelain throne, be patient. Definitely do not strain to have a BM, do not bear down to make something happen. Just sit and let nature take its course.

The reason I mention it is that straining on the toilet increases the pressure inside the chest, causing less blood flow to the heart; if done soon after heart surgery, it can make you feel dizzy or even pass out.

That's not a good way to get off the pot!

EXTRA CREDIT

Straining at bowel movements is a common cause of hemorrhoids. Bearing down without breathing out is called a **Valsalva maneuver**, and the increased pressure causes the veins near the anus to overfill with blood. It's a bit like having varicose veins of the back-side. Over time, these engorged veins can tear, causing inflammation and pain, even bleeding.

So, after heart surgery, you have more than one reason not to strain: avoiding passing out and avoiding hemorrhoids!

POD 4-5

Hopefully today you are feeling noticeably better. You no doubt still have soreness but less sharp pain.

Your breathing is stronger, less labored. Most patients still feel winded when walking at this point. We want to have you off the extra oxygen/nasal cannula before you go home, if possible. Usually an oxygen saturation >90% is safe and does not require extra oxygen — that is our goal.

You are walking by yourself, with or without the rolling walker. If you still need a walker for balance, don't fret — you are welcome to use it until your balance is nice and solid. If you have stairs at your house or apartment, a Physical Therapist can help you traverse a few stairs for confidence-building.

Hopefully your appetite is beginning to improve and you are getting a few more winks during the night.

GOING HOME

A lot of patients have mixed emotions about going home: they are happy to be improving and getting back home but also feel nervous about being away from professionals who know how to help.

Notwithstanding this natural nervousness, I want you to feel confident going home. I commit to you to not send you home until I believe you are ready, until I am convinced you will do well and be safe. I feel absolutely NO pressure from the hospital to send patients home in a certain timeframe. I would much rather keep you in the hospital an extra day or two, if it means you don't end up back in the hospital with a problem.

Your list of medications going home will be different than prior to surgery. Your nurse will go over your list of discharge medications to be sure you know what to take and when. Please let us know if you have questions about your medications.

A lot of patients ask about getting a hospital bed for the house. I'm not exactly opposed to that, but I usually recommend either sleeping in a recliner or using several pillows in bed if needed. Buying or renting a hospital bed is unnecessary for almost all patients.

Some patients ask me to arrange a Handicap Parking Permit for their car. I have never prescribed one. I want you walking. Park at the back of the parking lot, from my point of view! If you feel very strongly about it, see if your PCP would be willing to help you get one.

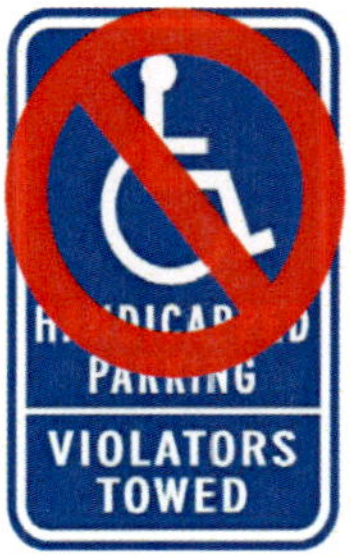

I recommend not driving a car for two weeks from

the day of your surgery. Other people may tell you longer but as your surgeon, I am saying that 2 weeks is a sufficient time-frame. Obviously, don't wreck! If you are going to wreck, wait a while longer. In all seriousness, though, after two weeks you can drive again as long as you are off pain medicines, since pain medicine could possibly impair your judgment or reaction time.

I recommend not doing any heavy lifting for two months from the day of surgery. The limit is 10 pounds, roughly the weight of a gallon of milk. Some Physical Therapists tell me this is overly restrictive, but I still think it is a good idea and easy to remember. The issue is not your heart but rather the breastbone aka sternum. We need to give the bone time to heal before stressing it. At two months, the bone will be 99% healed and you can't hurt it by lifting. Thus, at two months, you are cleared to do any kind of physical activity from my point of view, having no restrictions.

TAKE HOME POINTS

Don't drive for 2 weeks & don't lift for 2 months after CABG.

Along with lifting, I recommend not swinging a golf club for two months. Using a putter will not hurt your breastbone, so feel free to work on your putting as soon as you get home. In two months, go to the range and hit a bucket of balls. Ramp up from there and you can expect to get back to the course within another week or two.

If you have had robotic-assisted CABG, then you can engage in vigorous physical activity including lifting and golf as soon as you feel like it, that is, as soon as you feel comfortable and the motions do not worsen your soreness.

In terms of getting back to work, most patients can expect to be off work for 4-6 weeks after CABG. If you must lift over 10 pounds for work, then you need to be off two months. In contrast, if you work at a desk or from home, you can likely return to work earlier. It certainly is not unsafe to participate in a Zoom call or check email or speak with clients on the phone.

But be aware that most patients tire easily and have trouble working many hours in a row soon after CABG, just as they would after any major surgery. This tiredness and low stamina improve in time. Once you are ready for full duty, my office assistant will be happy to provide a Return-to-Work letter or form if needed.

TAKE HOME POINTS

Expect to Return to Work

In 2-4 weeks if working from home.

In 4-6 weeks if working at an office.

In 8 weeks if working outside or doing heavy lifting.

If you have had robotic-assisted CABG, you can expect to return to work earlier, often as early as 2 weeks.

It is convenient to have someone with you at home, whether your spouse or a family member. If no one can stay with you, that is okay – you definitely do not need someone there 24/7. It is helpful to have someone who is just a phone call away, who can check on you or help if problems arise, but they do not need to stay at your house.

I have a number of patients who live in rural areas far away from the nearest city, who do not have friends or family nearby. That is okay. You can get along safely by yourself, so do not fret if this is your situation.

AT HOME

Once home, it is important to stay active. **Keep walking** three times per day and increase the duration and distance of your walks. Keep working on your breathing exercises as well.

You may feel faint when you stand up; this is common after CABG.

Be sure you stand slowly and get your bearings prior to taking a first step. This phenomenon fades in time. If you are having a lot of trouble with this kind of dizziness/uneasiness, call my office and we'll advise adjustments to your medications; often, a contributing factor is blood pressure being slightly too low, so we'll back off on your BP medications. Be sure to stay hydrated, as dehydration can magnify the dizziness effect.

Watch for swelling of your feet or ankles. It is common to have *some* swelling, especially in the evenings, but if the swelling gets worse over a couple of days, call my office and let us know. Often, an extra dose or two of Lasix (a diuretic "water pill") is all that is needed to get rid of the swelling.

I invite you to visit my office after going home. Sometimes we can do this virtually with a video call. The visit is often within 1-2 weeks of discharge home. Please do not hesitate to call if any problems arise before or after your visit! PAs often help me see patients in the office.

TAKE HOME POINTS

Call any time with any questions & any problems.

I recommend **Cardiac Rehab** for almost all patients after CABG. Cardiac Rehab is like having a personal trainer, but the trainer is a medical professional who knows you had bypass surgery and can guide you in building strength while avoiding injury to your chest. I usually recommend starting cardiac rehab around 2 weeks after you go home. We'll plan to find the Cardiac Rehab program closest to your house.

Cardiac rehab is typically 3 days per week and each session lasts about an hour. You will likely meet other people who have recently had heart surgery; interacting with others going through a similar challenge will hopefully be encouraging for you. A Physical Therapist at Cardiac Rehab will guide you through activities designed to build your strength and mobility. Most patients have observable improvements in stamina after just a handful of sessions.

The full cardiac rehab program lasts up to 12 weeks. You may very well be feeling great before cardiac rehab ends; if you get bored with rehab because you are doing so well, feel free to graduate early and stop going. The program is there to help you over an extended period of time if you need it.

TAKE HOME POINTS

Cardiac Rehab will pump you up!

It is designed to speed you up, not slow you down.

Some patients are shy to ask about sexual activity but it is an issue of importance for many patients. Generally, sexual intercourse involves a similar exertion to climbing stairs, so if you can walk up 2 flights of stairs, you are physically safe to engage in intercourse. Of course, acrobatic feats or yoga-like contortions are to be discouraged for 2 months until your sternum heals. An understanding partner will ease the transition back to your full vigor.

To further clarify: Given that most patients have the capability of climbing 2 flights of stairs before leaving the hospital, you can return to sexual intercourse ad lib, meaning as soon as you feel like it.

However, do not be surprised if your level of interest in sexual activity seems diminished for a while, as this lull is common for many patients after CABG. Once your soreness resolves, your sleeping improves, your appetite returns, and your daily rhythm regains normalcy, your sexual activity will return to normal as well. Close communication with your partner can help you work through this process.

It is common for patients to have a depressed mood while recovering from CABG. It is a natural result of going through a major operation, having pain and shortness of breath, poor sleep and an emotional roller-coaster. Who would feel happy in the middle of all that?

Along with depressed mood, many patients experience lability of emotions, feeling happy one minute and sad the next, without any obvious reason. This is normal and nothing to be embarassed about.

Larry King, the late television personality, wrote of his own experience after CABG:

> **"I found that after the surgery you go through a period where you'll find yourself crying for no apparent reason. Just burst into tears... happened to me on a plane down to Miami. Just — boom! I'm sitting there reading the airline magazine and suddenly I'm weeping. Guy in the next seat thought I'd lost my mind..."** [13]

Don't feel bad if your emotions seem difficult to control. As you heal and recover, your personality and emotions will return to normal.

I usually ask you to see your cardiologist within a month after your operation. I am happy for your cardiologist to adjust your medicines as he or she sees fit. Your cardiologist will likely want to see you once or twice per year on an ongoing basis.

Long-term, I usually see my CABG patients as needed and do not ask you to automatically come to my office every year. I will "release you to the wild" and expect that you will do very well for many years. Of course please call if any problems arise. And please feel free to drop in if you are near the office, as I am always happy to see my patients "in real life;" it is quite satisfying to me as a surgeon to know you are doing well.

TAKE HOME POINTS

Your emotions will likely roam far & wide.

Your romantic interest may range from none to small.

Your energy may seem to wander & hide.

God will strengthen you through it all.

A GOOD RESOLUTION

If you've never read a thinly-veiled epilogue before, today is your lucky day.

Anonymous

For hundreds if not thousands of years, the heart has been considered the seat of human consciousness and the soul.

In ancient Egypt, regulations for embalming required the heart to be maintained in place, not removed with the other organs. It was considered the most sacred part of a man.

The Bible advises "Guard your heart, for it is the well-spring of life" (Proverbs 4:23).

Modern science would suggest consciousness resides somewhere in the brain, and while the exact "location" of the soul remains elusive, it doesn't seem to be inside the chambers of the heart. But even if bereft of consciousness and soul, the heart maintains a mystique not afforded any other part of the body.

Leviticus 17:11 reads, "The life of the creature is in the blood." No biologist can explain the mysterious nature of life, but theologically and practically, we cannot live without blood. This precious blood does not circulate without the heart. The heart gives motion to life, and from generation to generation, the heart remains of inestimable worth to each of us and all of us.

Its worth works its way deep into our feelings and language: adolescents emerging into adulthood quickly learn the happy weight of the symbols "I ❤ U." At all ages, the heart commands a front-and-center role in the affairs of love. When words from the mind fail to express our deepest emotions and longings, the heart succeeds.

Central to our bodies, central to our lives, central to our love. The heart is central to who we are. God has given each of us a great gift in giving us our heart.

Will a viable artificial heart ever be made? Perhaps. Who can know the future except God Himself? There are artificial hearts which have been used but none works as well as one would hope. There are pesky problems of bleeding and blood clots, not to mention mechanical components which break down and fail. Nothing that lasts more than 7 or 8 years, let alone 70 or 80! Like the blood it moves, the natural human heart so far has defied human engineering. Indeed, it defies our understanding.

It looks like muscle and connective tissue, but I am suspicious it is something more. I suspect it is more than just a collection of cells, more than simply a collection of molecules and chemical bonds. What else links and transcends mind, body and spirit?

I continue to be amazed by the heart, though I have seen and touched thousands of them. As you now know, the heart is in a class by itself: sensitive to our thoughts, nervous input, and hormones but capable of beating without them. Composed of special cells which work constantly but never fatigue, cells acting individually like muscles and collectively like nerves. Working every moment of your life, never stopping to rest, never letting you down.

Your heart is unlike anything else.

It is my privilege to be a heart surgeon. I wish everyone could see the heart as I see it, to have the honor of holding a heart in his or her hands.

To see the beauty of its motion, the elegance of its design. To feel the amazement of it stopping, the glory of it starting again. To experience the magnificence of something which has no equal.

As you continue on your journey of life, I hope you think of your heart more than you did before. I hope you appreciate it more. Care for it more. ❤ it more.

With so much at stake, I'm willing to guess this is a challenging time for you. I would encourage you that in the end, good can come from adversity. Remember the pediatrician who said we needed to talk about my daughter, Jane Maddy?

LETS GET PERSONAL

He went on to say that she has a severe genetic syndrome. That the doctors sent some tests off but my wife and I should take her home because she would die in the next few days. Talk about a shocking situation! I did not see how it could be true. But several experts saw her and said the same thing.

My wife and I took her to our church at 4 days old, and hundreds of people prayed for her. My wife and I chose to trust God, realizing she is His daughter, and she is in His hands.

By God's grace, her genetic tests were found to be normal several days later. She has all the outward signs of the syndrome, but none of the inner effects. Now, several years later, she is alive and doing well. She has challenges, and our family is grateful for the strengthening of our faith as we see her overcome them. We are grateful for her life, grateful for each day.

I know her precious life matters to God. And I look forward to seeing how she will impact this world, because of her special story.

By God's grace, CABG will help you live a full life. Your heart will be better, though you will bear a scar, the outward sign of your difficult challenge. Going through it all is tough, but your special story will have a new chapter — a significant and profound one.

No matter what the future holds, know that you matter to God and you are in His hands. May He give you strength and grace today and in the days ahead!

GLOSSARY

Aberrant: different from normal, as in, an aberrant artery is an artery with an unusual location or course.

ABG: short for Arterial Blood Gas, a blood test taken from an artery used to determine oxygen and carbon dioxide levels.

Ablation: procedure designed to restore a normal heart rhythm, often as therapy for atrial fibrillation. A MAZE is a form of ablation performed as part of a surgical operation.

ACE inhibitor: short for Angiotensin-Converting-Enzyme inhibitor, a medication which relaxes arteries, causing a lowering of blood pressure.

ACS: short for Acute Coronary Syndrome, a set of signs and symptoms related to impaired coronary blood flow and myocardial damage.

Acute: a disease or condition recent in onset or having a short duration.

Acute MI: short for Acute Myocardial Infarction, a fresh or recent heart attack.

Ad lib: short for ad libitum, a Latin phrase meaning "as you desire."

AED: short for Automated External Defibrillator, a portable electrical device which delivers an electric shock to treat ventricular fibrillation and restore a normal heart rhythm. Designed to be used by a person without medical training and often found at public places such as a library or sporting venue.

Aerobic exercise: physical exercise involving rhythmic, continuous motions for a sustained period of time, designed to raise the heart rate. The term "aerobics" was coined by Dr. Kenneth Cooper in his book Aerobics, first published in 1968.

Afib: short for Atrial Fibrillation.

AICD: short for Automated Implantable Cardioverter-Defibrillator, a medical device placed beneath the skin, capable of detecting and treating abnormal heart rhythms.

Ambulate: fancy medical word for walking.

Anaerobic metabolism: method of energy (ATP) production which occurs in the absence of oxygen; roughly 15-30 times less efficient than aerobic metabolism.

Analgesic: medication used to reduce pain.

Anastomosis: a surgical connection made between two structures, such as blood vessels.

Anemia: condition of low level of red blood cells in the blood.

Aneurysm: an enlarged portion of a blood vessel. Can also rarely refer to a chamber of the heart. Typically the wall of an aneurysm is thinner than normal and bulges out, making it more likely to tear or rupture than a normal artery.

Angina pectoris: chest discomfort which occurs due to impaired blood flow and oxygen delivery to the heart muscle. Angina classically begins with exertion and resolves with rest.

Angiogram: a movie-like sequence of x-ray images showing blood vessels filled by contrast dye.

Angioplasty: a procedure in which a balloon is inflated inside an artery to forcefully open a blockage. The balloon pushes plaque against the walls of the artery and enlarges the artery slightly.

Anoxia: absence of oxygen.

Anticoagulant: a medication which reduces the clotting capacity of the blood. Commonly called a blood thinner, although anticoagulants do not affect the viscosity of blood to an appreciable extent.

Antiplatelet agent: a medication which reduces the activation or "stickiness" of platelets, thereby decreasing the chance of thrombus formation and occlusion of a blood vessel or stent.

Aorta: the main artery carrying blood from the heart to the tissues of the body. The aorta is the largest artery in the body.

Aortic Insufficiency: abbreviated AI; synonymous with aortic regurgitation. Involves blood moving in reverse direction back into the heart during diastole, because the aortic valve is not closing properly.

Arrhythmia: abnormal rhythm of the heart; synonymous with dysrhythmia.

Arteriosclerosis: "hardening of the arteries." Disease of arteries involving loss of elasticity, which tends to become more common with advancing age.

ASAP: short for As Soon As Possible.

Ascending aorta: the first portion of the aorta, which begins at the aortic annulus and ends at the aortic arch.

Asymptomatic: not having or causing symptoms.

Asystole: cessation of the electrical activity of the heart. Results in a "flat line" on an EKG tracing, as commonly shown in movies to allude to a character's death.

Atherectomy: a procedure designed to cut through hardened, calcified blockages in an artery using a rotating blade, much like a tiny Roto-Rooter. A highly-specialized procedure, typically performed only in high-volume centers by select interventional cardiologists.

Atherosclerosis: disease of arteries involving build-up of fatty deposits and plaque.

Atrial fibrillation: aka afib; an abnormal heart rhythm involving rapid and chaotic electrical activity in the atrial chambers of the heart; it amounts to a tremorous shaking of the atria. Results in a so-called "irregularly irregular" rhythm on EKG.

Atrial Septal Defect: abbreviated ASD; a defect in the interatrial septum. Much like a PFO but larger, allowing blood to mix between atria. If a patient develops symptoms, an ASD may require closure.

Atrium: from Latin root *atria* meaning central court; chamber which receives blood and channels it to a ventricle. The right atrium receives blood from the

IVC and SVC, channeling it to the right ventricle. The left atrium receives blood from the pulmonary veins, channeling it to the left ventricle.

Auscultation: process of listening to internal organs of the body, usually with a stethoscope.

AV block: impairment or interruption of conduction of electrical impulses from the atria to the ventricles. Defined in degrees: first, second or third (complete).

AV node: a special collection of cells which transmit electrical impulses from the atria to the ventricles.

AVR: short for Aortic Valve Replacement, an operation involving removal of a diseased aortic valve and insertion of a new valve. Historically the most common operation performed on a heart valve. SAVR refers to Surgical AVR, whereas TAVR refers to Transcatheter AVR.

BAV: short for Balloon Aortic Valvuloplasty. A percutaneous procedure whereby a balloon is inflated inside a tight aortic valve to forcefully open it. Effective in treating aortic stenosis but has a temporary effect, usually lasting only weeks to perhaps months. BAV may also less commonly refer to a bicuspid aortic valve.

Beta-blocker: a medication which reduces the activity of adrenaline by binding to Beta receptors of cells of the myocardium, blood vessels and sympathetic nervous system. A Beta-blocker lowers the blood pressure and heart rate. Metoprolol is a commonly-used example.

Bicuspid Aortic Valve: an abnormal aortic valve which has only two moving parts (leaflets, or cusps) instead of the usual three. The most common congenital abnormality of the heart, affecting 2% of the population.

BID: short for Latin phrase *bis in die* meaning twice per day.

Bifurcation: fancy medical term for branching point. Blockages in arteries often occur at a bifurcation.

Blood pressure: Force (per unit area) exerted by the blood within arteries, which is produced by contraction of the heart muscle. Commonly measured at the level of the brachial artery in the arm just above the elbow. Typically given in mmHg, which is the height in millimeters a column of Mercury would rise when pushed by that pressure.

BMI: short for Body Mass Index, a metric comparing a person's body weight to height. Calculated by dividing a person's weight (in kg) by the person's height (in meters) squared. A normal BMI is 20-25 kg/m2, overweight 25-30 kg/m2 and obese >30 kg/m2.

BNP : short for B-type Natriuretic Peptide, a protein produced by cells in the heart in response to dilation of the heart. It is sometimes called Brain Natriuretic Peptide, because it was first found in the brain, but it is made in the heart. Used as a blood test to help gauge the severity of heart failure.

Board-Certified: designation of a physician who has demonstrated mastery of knowledge and skill in a field of medicine or surgery, as determined by a national Board. Board-certification is voluntary and not a legal requirement for practicing medicine or surgery in the USA; however, hospitals may require physicians to maintain Board-certification in order to practice at their facility. The American Board of Thoracic Surgery provides certification for cardiac surgeons.

Bovine: related to a cow or cattle.

Brachytherapy: technique in which a tiny radiation source is placed within a coronary artery, typically to treat in-stent re-stenosis. Brachytherapy is a fairly rare technique and does not have a role in the treatment of patients at many programs.

Bradycardia: a slow heart rate, generally less than 60 beats per minute, or a rate that is slower than expected for a patient's age, condition or activity level.

Bruit: pronounced BRU-ee; a sound made by turbulent blood flow within a blood vessel, possibly due to a blockage. A classic source of a bruit is the carotid arteries.

Bundle of His: specialized muscle cells in the interventricular septum which transmit electrical signals from the AV node to the ventricles. Discovered by Dr. Wilhelm His (pronounced hiss) in 1893.

Bundle Branch Block: a disorder of the heart's electrical signaling in which signals traveling through the left or right bundle branches are impaired; this slowing or blocking of signals results in one ventricle contracting before the other.

CABG: pronounced CABB-age; aka Coronary Artery Bypass Grafting. Operation designed to provide additional pathways for blood to flow to the myocardium. Most common heart operation in the USA.

CAD: pronounced C-A-D; aka Coronary Artery Disease. Build-up of plaque within the arteries of the heart, leading to blockage of blood flood and impaired delivery of oxygen to the heart muscle.

Calcium-channel blocker: medication which slows the passage of calcium into muscle cells of blood vessels and the heart. Less calcium means less vigorous contraction, so the blood pressure goes down.

Cannula: plastic tube placed into a blood vessel or the heart.

Capillaries: tiny blood vessels within tissues which allow for exchange of oxygen and carbon dioxide.

Cardiac: fancy medical word which means having to do with the heart.

Cardiac arrest: cessation of effective motion of the heart.

Cardiac catheterization: medical procedure where a small catheter is guided from an artery in the groin or wrist into the arteries of the heart; used to determine anatomic details and diagnose problems such as CAD.

Cardiac enzymes: chemicals present in heart muscle cells which do not normally circulate in the bloodstream. Injury to heart muscle cells results in release of the enzymes, such that they can be detected in the blood. Troponin is a cardiac enzyme.

Cardiac Output: the amount of blood pumped by the heart in one minute, usually around 5 liters for an adult. If the heart is weakened and the EF is low, cardiac output may be reduced. If the cardiac output is less than what the body tissues need, the condition is known as heart failure.

Cardiac Rehab: exercise and support program designed to help patients recover after heart surgery, similar to going to a gym to work with a private trainer. But the Cardiac Rehab specialist knows what exercises are safe to do after surgery and can make assessments of heart rate and blood pressure. Typically done 3 days per week for 12 weeks.

Cardiogenic shock: inadequate blood flow to body organs due to sudden impairment in heart function, often due to heart attack. Has a high risk of death unless promptly relieved.

Cardiologist: a medical doctor who specializes in caring for the heart.

Cardiomegaly: an enlarged heart. The most common cause of cardiomegaly is dilated cardiomyopathy.

Cardiomyopathy: from Greek, literal translation is "heart muscle suffering." A disorder involving impaired function of the heart.

Cardiopulmonary bypass: technology used to replace the function of heart and lungs; aka the heart-lung machine.

Cardioversion: a procedure designed to convert an abnormal heart rhythm to a normal rhythm using an electrical shock. Cardioversion differs from defibrillation in that cardioversion syncs with the patients rhythm to deliver the shock at a specific point in the cardiac cycle, whereas defibrillation delivers the shock at a random time, since there is not rhythmicity to ventricular fibrillation to coordinate the timing.

Carotid artery: major artery in the neck on both right and left sides supplying blood to the brain.

Carotid endarterectomy: operation designed to remove plaque from a carotid artery, thereby reducing the risk of stroke.

Catheter: a small tube, usually made of plastic, inserted into a part of the body.

Chest tube: a plastic tube which drains fluid, blood or air from the chest, into a collection chamber. At least one chest tube is inserted as part of every heart surgery, preventing blood from accumulating around the heart after operation. The tube is removed in the patient's room once it is not needed anymore.

CHF: see Congestive Heart Failure.

Cholesterol: a fatty chemical produced by animal cells, needed for cell membranes.

Circulator nurse: a Registered Nurse who attends to the patient and materials during an operation and records documentation of OR events.

Circumflex Artery: coronary artery arising from the Left Main, serving the left side and part of the back of the heart.

Claudication: pain, discomfort or tiredness of the legs which occurs with walking and resolves with rest. May indicate blockages in the arteries of the pelvis or legs.

Coagulation: fancy medical term for clotting of blood, the process by which blood changes from a liquid to a gel and ultimately a semi-solid.

Code brown: slang term used when a patient did not make it to the bathroom in time for #2.

Coenzyme Q10: chemical in the body's cells which helps facilitate energy production. Likely has an underappreciated role in cellular repair and the regulation of inflammation.

Collateral arteries: small pathways which connect major arteries and allow some flow of blood when one of the arteries is occluded (completely blocked).

Co-morbidity: a condition or disease which co-exists with the condition of primary interest.

Complete heart block: aka third-degree atrioventricular block. Damage to the AV node leads to obstruction of electrical signals from the atria to ventricles. May require a pacemaker to address.

Conduit: the blood vessel used as a new pathway for blood flow with bypass surgery.

Congenital: a condition present at birth. A congenital heart defect is an abnormality of the heart present at birth. The most common congenital heart defect is a bicuspid aortic valve.

Congestive heart failure: aka CHF. A condition in which the heart is unable to pump out all of the blood returning to it, so blood and fluids accumulate in other tissues, leading to congestion. If the right side of the heart "fails," blood backs up into the liver and lower body, causing swelling; if the left heart "fails," blood backs up into the lungs, causing shortness of breath.

COPD: short for Chronic Obstructive Pulmonary Disease. A lung disease, most commonly caused by smoking cigarettes, characterized by poor air flow and shortness of breath.

Coronary artery: from Latin root *corona* meaning "crown." An artery supplying blood to the heart.

Coronary Heart Disease: same thing as CAD.

Coronary sinus: the main vein draining blood from the heart muscle. Empties into the right atrium.

CPAP: short for Continuous Positive Airway Pressure. A form of ventilation where a machine maintains air pressure inside the patient's airway above atmospheric pressure. Commonly used to treat obstructive sleep apnea.

CPR: short for CardioPulmonary Resuscitation. Used when a person's heart has stopped beating, aka cardiac arrest. Involves chest compressions to compress the heart from the outside and maintain circulation of blood, to keep the person alive until more advanced help can be delivered or the heart begins to beat again on its own.

CT scan: short for Computed Tomography, aka CAT scan (Computed Axial Tomography). Produces images of internal anatomy based on a series of closely spaced x-rays which are compiled by computer. Can be done with contrast given into a vein or swallowed by mouth or without any contrast. Contrast helps anatomic details be more accurately seen.

Cusp: flap of tissue which moves in a heart valve – the part actually opening and closing. A normal aortic valve has 3 cusps and the mitral valve 2 cusps.

CVA: short for CerebroVascular Accident aka stroke. Damage to the brain which results from inadequate blood flow, equivalent to a heart attack. May be due to impaired blood flow (ischemic stroke) or due to bleeding (hemorrhagic stroke).

CXR: short for Chest X-Ray, which shows structures in the chest and may show certain pathology such as fluid around the lungs (pleural effusion). Fine details of small structures cannot be seen on a CXR.

Cyanosis: a bluish coloration of skin or tissues due to reduced oxygen content of the blood.

Cyclo-oxygenase: aka COX, an enzyme which helps form prostaglandins; NSAIDs such as Aspirin block the action of COX, thereby reducing inflammation and reducing activation/stickiness of platelets.

DAPT: short for Dual Anti-Platelet Therapy, which involves taking two medicines to inhibit platelet function, in order to avoid thrombosis inside a fresh stent. Aspirin and Plavix are often used.

Debridement: pronounced duh-BREED-mint; removal of diseased tissue or foreign material by surgical means.

Decompensated heart failure: inadequate pumping of the heart which has led to sudden worsening of fluid retention and swelling, requiring prompt medical attention.

Decompress: reduce the pressure.

Defibrillator: a device which delivers an electric shock in order to restore a normal heart rhythm. Typically used to treat ventricular fibrillation. May be external to the body (AED) or placed inside the body (AICD).

DES: short for Drug-Eluting Stent, a small metal tube designed to hold a blockage open in a coronary artery. The stent features a polymer coating on its inner surface which releases tiny amounts of a drug to help prevent overgrowth of cells within the stent.

Diabetes mellitus: a disease involving abnormal regulation of insulin, leading to excess levels of sugar in the bloodstream.

Diaphoresis: fancy medical word for excessive sweating.

Diastole: the time period during which the heart muscle relaxes. This corresponds to the diastolic blood pressure, when the arteries in the body also relax slightly and the blood pressure lowers.

Diastolic blood pressure: the lowest blood pressure measured in the arteries, which occurs when the heart is in the relaxation or filling phase of the cardiac cycle. A common BP reading is 120/80 mmHg, where 80 mmHg is the diastolic pressure.

Diffuse: to move from an area of high

concentration to lower concentration.

Dilatation: condition of being enlarged beyond normal dimension, becoming dilated.

Dilated: condition of being larger or more open than normal.

Dilated cardiomyopathy: a condition in which the heart muscle is enlarged, or dilated, leading to thinning and impaired function.

Distal: farther from a point of reference; in terms of arteries, refers to a portion of the artery farther from its origin. The term is also used to describe the site of connection of a conduit to a coronary artery during CABG, as in, "I sewed the LIMA to the distal."

Diuretic: a medication which causes an increase in the production and passage of urine. Lasix is a common diuretic (not to be confused with LASIK, which is a procedure performed on the eyes).

DNR: short for Do Not Resuscitate, an order which lets hospital personnel know if the patient's heart stops, they should not attempt to make it beat again – i.e., CPR will not be performed. In general, if a DNR order is in place prior to operation, it must be suspended for heart surgery, since the heart will be stopped intentionally.

Door-to-balloon: term used to describe the time from presentation of a STEMI patient at the "door" of the ER to inflation of the balloon during angioplasty. A short door-to-balloon time implies excellent coordination of care.

Doppler ultrasound: imaging technology which uses sound waves to assess the motion of the heart and blood flow.

Dressler's syndrome: inflammation of the pericardium, often due to an immune response after a heart attack or heart surgery.

Dropsy: outdated synonym for edema.

DVT: short for Deep Vein Thrombosis, a blood clot which forms in a vein deep in the leg, often due to reduced physical activity or immobilization. May result in pain or swelling in the leg or may not cause obvious symptoms. A DVT can move to the lungs, becoming a pulmonary embolism.

Dysrhythmia: abnormal heart beat; aka arrhythmia.

Dyspnea: fancy medical word for shortness of breath. Often phrased as dyspnea on exertion = shortness of breath when physically active.

ECG: short for ElectroCardioGram; see EKG.

Echocardiogram: an ultrasound of the heart. First named "ultrasound cardiography" by echo pioneer Dr. Inge Edler. Provides images of the heart in motion, including the ventricular muscle and the heart valves. May be through the skin (TTE) or down the esophagus (TEE).

ECMO: short for ExtraCorporeal Membrane Oxygenation, pronounced ECK-mo. Complex machine which works like the heart-lung machine to pump blood and put oxygen in the blood, designed to function outside the Operating Room. Used on a temporary basis when the heart and/or lungs are unable to support life. The technology involves risks of complications such as bleeding and infection but can be life-saving for certain patients. Rarely used (rarely needed) in association with heart bypass surgery, except when the heart works very poorly at the end of an operation.

Ectopic heartbeat: type of dysrhythmia where the ventricles contract slightly too early or slightly too late, creating an extra beat or a dropped beat and disrupting the regularity of the rhythm. Usually harmless and can be part of normal heart function.

Edema: pronounced eh-DEE-ma. Swelling of body tissues due to accumulation of fluid. Commonly affects the feet and ankles.

EEG: short for ElectroEncephaloGram. Measures and records electrical activity of the brain. Not used commonly for heart surgery patients, and not to be confused with EKG or TEE.

Ejection Fraction: aka EF. The fraction of blood ejected from the heart with each contraction, stated as a percentage. A normal EF is 60%; this means that 40% of the blood stays within the heart during each contraction and the heart is never empty, no matter how fast it beats. Can refer to either the Left Ventricular EF (LVEF) or the Right Ventricular EF (RVEF); if not specified, EF is assumed to mean LVEF.

EKG: short for ElectroKardioGramm. A tracing of the electric potentials of the heart, created using several leads in contact with the skin.

Electrolyte: a chemical with ions dissolved in a fluid such as water; in the body usually refers to salts, acids and bases needed for metabolic regulation.

Embolism: lodging of a piece of material inside a blood vessel; often, the material is a blood clot. Though rare, an embolism to a coronary artery could cause a heart attack. An embolism to the brain could cause a stroke. During heart surgery, care is taken to avoid an air embolism, a condition where air from the heart-lung machine obstructs a blood vessel — who knew that air could stop the flow of blood?!

Emphysema: lung disease characterized by disruption of alveoli such that gas exchange is impaired. Basically, the microscopic air sacs become large, thereby moving the oxygen farther from the capillaries nearby and making it harder for carbon dioxide to move out of the air sacs when the person breathes out. Some forms of emphysema are associated with cigarette smoking.

EMS: short for Emergency Medical Services, refers to ambulance and paramedic service. An EMT is an Emergency Medical Technician and provides care as part of EMS. A paramedic has additional training and expertise.

Endarterectomy: surgical removal of plaque from an artery. Not usually performed during CABG, since a new pathway around the plaque is provided and the plaque is not disturbed; endarterectomy is commonly performed for plaque in the carotid arteries.

Endocarditis: inflammation of the inner layer of the heart, the endocardium. Usually due to a bacterial infection.

Endocardium: the innermost layer of cells, or lining, within the heart. The endocardium is continuous with the endothelium of the arteries and veins of the body.

Endothelium: single layer of cells which line all blood vessels in the body and is contiguous with the endocardium in the heart. The endothelial layer of the circulatory system is in direct contact with blood.

Enema: pronounced N-eh-muh. Injection of fluid into the rectum designed to prompt evacuation of the bowels. Not to be confused with edema.

Enzyme: a chemical able to speed up biochemical reactions in the body.

EP: short for ElectroPhysiologist, a cardiologist who specializes in the treatment of abnormal heart rhythms.

Epicardium: a thin film of cells which covers the outer surface of heart tissues.

Epinephrine: aka adrenaline. Hormone made by the adrenal gland. Epinephrine has many actions in numerous tissues in the body, including increasing the heart rate and strength of heart muscle contraction.

Erythema: fancy medical word for redness.

Erythrocyte: red blood cell which contains hemoglobin and transports oxygen in the blood.

Essential Hypertension: aka primary hypertension. Refers to blood pressure > 120/80 mmHg without another medical cause.

ET Tube: short for EndoTracheal Tube. A plastic tube placed through the mouth into the trachea to allow for breathing during a general anesthetic and/or to facilitate use of a mechanical ventilator (breathing machine). If an ETT is not used in these situations, air can too easily move into the esophagus and stomach rather than the trachea and lungs.

Etiology: the study of the cause of a disease.

EVH: short for Endoscopic Vein Harvest, a method to extract a vein from the leg for use in CABG using a video camera and small incisions.

Exertion: physical use of energy, resulting in motion.

Extubate: to remove a patient's breathing tube.

Familial Hypercholesterolemia: genetic disorder characterized by LDL dysfunction, leading to high levels of cholesterol in the blood.

Fellow: a doctor in an advanced and specialized phase of training known as fellowship, having completed internship and residency.

Femoral artery: large artery coursing not far from the femur bone in the groin, providing blood to the leg.

Fibrillation: a cardiac dysrhythmia characterized by disorderly, chaotic quivering of myocardium. Can affect the atria or ventricles. Atrial fibrillation is not generally life-threatening and may resolve on its own, but ventricular fibrillation is usually fatal if not promptly corrected. A defibrillator detects ventricular fibrillation and delivers an electrical impulse in order to convert the fibrillation to a regular rhythm, but the device will not take action when sensing atrial fibrillation since impulse delivery is not needed.

Fibrosis: fancy medical word for scarring.

Flutter: a cardiac dysrhythmia characterized by rapid but abbreviated contractions of the heart. Flutter is usually slightly more organized than fibrillation.

Foley catheter: plastic tube inserted through the urethra into the bladder. Usually used during long operations or when a patient cannot get out of bed to urinate.

Ganglia: groups of nerve cells located outside the central nervous system.

General anesthetic: medication given to achieve unconsciousness so that a patient does not experience awareness or pain during an operation.

H&P: short for History and Physical, the parts of a doctor-patient interaction which include gathering information about patient symptoms and examination.

Harvest: to move a blood vessel out of its normal location so it can be used as a bypass graft.

HDL: short for High Density Lipoprotein, molecule which transports cholesterol away from cells in the body to the liver.

Heart attack: aka myocardial infarction. Refers to damage to heart muscle cells due to inadequate blood flow and delivery of oxygen through the coronary arteries.

Heart block: interruption of the conduction of electrical signals from the atria to the ventricles.

Heart failure: inability of the heart to pump an adequate volume of blood. The term does not refer to a literal, complete loss of the function of the heart, as this would result in death.

Heart-lung machine: machine used during heart surgery which pumps the blood (assuming the function of the heart) and allows gas exchange (puts oxygen in the blood and takes carbon dioxide out, assuming the function of the lungs). Used for On-Pump CABG and valve operations, so that the patient's heart can be stopped and remain still for accurate placement of sutures. The machine is controlled by a perfusionist.

Hematoma: a collection of blood in tissues, like a three-dimensional bruise.

Hemoglobin: protein inside red blood cells which binds oxygen and carbon dioxide, changing color depending on its binding or non-binding to oxygen.

Hemoglobin A1c: form of hemoglobin chemically linked to a sugar molecule. Used as a blood test to gauge the average blood sugar levels over a three-month period of time. Abbreviated as HbA1c.

Hemorrhage: fancy medical word for bleeding.

Hemorrhoids: engorged and inflamed veins near the anus.

Heparin: a commonly-used anticoagulant, or so-called blood thinner. Used in high dosage to prevent blood clotting inside the heart-lung machine and used in small doses to prevent blood clots in hospitalized patients. Heparin is not absorbed by the bowels so there is no pill form and it must be given by injection. Discovered in 1916 from liver tissue of dogs, most heparin now comes from cow lungs or pig intestines. Yes, you cannot make this stuff up (Notice the pun? There is no known way to synthesize heparin)!

Hibernating myocardium: areas of heart muscle affected by lack of oxygen during a heart attack which can return to normal function if blood flow is restored. I think of it as weak heart muscle which can be strong again if woken up by better blood flow.

Holter monitor: portable device invented by physicist Norman Holter, used to monitor a patient's heart rate and rhythm for 24 hours or more.

Hormone: a chemical produced in one body tissue which acts on another (distant) tissue or organ in the body.

Hospitalist: medical doctor who specializes in providing care to patients admitted to the hospital.

Hypercholesterolemia: elevated levels of cholesterol in the bloodstream. Thought to contribute to CAD and other diseases. Commonly treated by diet and lifestyle modification and/or statin medications.

Hyperdynamic: refers to ventricular function which is above normal with EF >70%.

Hypertension: aka high blood pressure. A condition characterized by an elevated force of blood pushing against the body's arterial walls. Commonly treated by diet, exercise, and anti-hypertensive medications.

Hypertrophic Obstructive Cardiomyopathy: abbreviated HOCM, pronounced HO-kum. Aka IHSS or Idiopathic Hypertrophic Subaortic Stenosis. A disorder involving overgrowth of the muscle of the septum between the ventricles; the muscle bulges beneath the aortic valve, interfering with movement of blood out of the heart.

Hypertrophy: fancy medical word for excessive thickness of the heart muscle. The heart muscle is thicker not because new cells have been added; rather, the muscle cells become larger.

Hypotension: low blood pressure.

Hypoxia: low oxygen levels in body tissues.

IABP: short for Intra-Aortic Balloon Pump. Device inserted through an artery in the groin which inflates inside the aorta, improving blood flow in the coronary arteries. Can be useful for cases of severe weakness of the heart after heart surgery; an Impella is also commonly used for this contingency.

Iatrogenic: caused by a physician or other health-care provider.

ICD: short for Implantable Cardioverter Defibrillator; see AICD.

ICU: short for Intensive Care Unit. Area of hospital providing continuous patient care and advanced life support technologies. Sometimes called MICU for Medical ICU and SICU for Surgical ICU.

Idiopathic: has no known cause or the cause has not been identified. It's the fancy word doctors use when they don't want to admit, I don't know!

IHSS: short for Idiopathic Hypertrophic Subaortic Stenosis; see Hypertrophic Obstructive Cardiomyopathy.

Ileus: decreased propulsive action of the intestines, which is often associated with bloating and distention of the abdomen. I think of it as the equivalent of the bowels going to sleep so that foodstuffs (stool) are not pushed downstream. Can be due to severe illness or as a response to major surgery. If a patient experiences nausea, vomiting, abdominal pain and distention after surgery, the diagnosis may be ileus. Typically with a post-op ileus, "tincture of time" is the only therapy needed; in severe cases, an NG tube may be placed to decompress the stomach.

Impella: brand name of a medical device which works like a pump to move blood out of the heart, when the heart is severely weak. An Impella is usually placed through the skin (percutaneously) via an artery in the groin or near the collar-bone and guided into position within the heart. It provides temporary support for several days or weeks until the heart is stronger.

Incise: to make a cut with a sharp surgical instrument.

Incompetent valve: aka regurgitant or insufficient valve. Term refers to a valve which does not close properly and allows blood to flow the wrong direction within the heart.

Infarction: death (necrosis) of cells due to inadequate blood flow.

Infective endocarditis: infection of the inner lining of the heart, the endocardium, often involving the heart valves. Can be caused by bacteria which travel through the bloodstream from another site of infection and stick to the endocardium.

Inflammation: complex biologic response of the body to infection, damage or irritation. Characterized by redness, warmth, swelling, pain and loss of function of the affected body part.

Inotrope: medication which increases the force of contraction of the myocardium.

Inpatient: fancy medical word used to describe a test or procedure performed with a patient admitted to the hospital.

Insufficiency: aka regurgitation. Refers to inadequate closing of a heart valve and blood moving backward through the valve; see Aortic Insufficiency and Mitral Regurgitation.

Intensivist: a medical doctor specializing in intensive care, taking care of patients in an ICU. Not to be confused with Internist.

Intern: a medical doctor training in his or her first year after graduating medical school. If you are in the hospital and an intern is taking care of you, drop this book and run to the nearest exit! Just kidding. Every doctor has to learn somewhere. Interns are overseen by attending physicians. An intern is also known as a first-year Resident or R1.

Internist: a medical doctor who specializes in the field of Internal Medicine. Like a pediatrician for adults — but not called an Adultist or Grownupatrician for unclear reasons. Not to be confused with an Intern.

Intima: the innermost lining of a blood vessel. The endothelium is part of the intima.

Intubate: to insert a breathing tube, through the mouth and into the trachea. An intubated patient is one with a breathing tube (ETT) in place.

Ion: when the "boyfriend" comes by the house before a date with my daughter, I let him know I've got an Ion (him). Is anyone reading this? Anyway, an ion is more traditionally described as a positively or negatively charged particle.

IS: short for Incentive Spirometer (or Spirometry), a device used to focus and strengthen a patient's breathing after operation. Often has a gauge which moves up to help the patient focus his or her effort. Air is breathed in through the spirometer, as opposed to a PEP device, where air is blown out.

Ischemia: a restriction or impairment in blood supply to tissues, causing insufficient oxygen delivery for cellular metabolism.

Ischemic heart disease: aka CAD.

iso-CABG: term describing a heart operation where bypasses are performed and no other major change to the heart is made, such as valve replacement. The iso-CABG operation is one of the most heavily studied and scrutinized operations in the history of surgery.

IV: short for IntraVenous, refers to something inside a vein. In common usage, an "IV" is a small catheter placed inside a vein, used to give medications and to draw blood for lab tests.

IVC: short for Inferior Vena Cava, the large vein which drains blood from the lower body to the right atrium of the heart.

IVUS: short for IntraVascular UltraSound, a medical technology which can be used as part of a cardiac cath to assess arteries for blockages using sound waves.

JCAHO: The Joint Commission on Accreditation of Healthcare Organizations, now called simply The Joint Commission. A non-profit organization which visits hospitals to assess quality and insure standards of care. Hospital administrators act like it is Homeland Security, the US Supreme Court and the papacy rolled into one organization.

LAA: short for Left Atrial Appendage. An outpouching of the left atrium, where blood clots tend to form in cases of afib.

Lactic acid: aka lactate. Organic acid which results from cellular metabolism.

LAD: short for Left Anterior Descending, pronounced L.A.D. The major coronary artery on the front of the heart. Colloquially called the "widowmaker" due to a high risk of death when acutely occluded.

LDL: short for Low Density Lipoprotein, a molecule which transports cholesterol to body cells. It is desirable to have a low level of LDL in the blood, as a low LDL level is associated with reduced risk of CAD.

Leaflets: thin, flexible pieces of tissue which make up the moving parts of a heart valve; also called cusps.

Left atrium: from Latin *atrium meaning* "entry hall or central court;" the heart chamber blood enters when returning from the lungs.

LHC: short for Left Heart Catheterization, a procedure performed by an interventional cardiologist to evaluate coronary anatomy and CAD.

Ligate: to tie or close off with suture.

LIMA: short for Left Internal Mammary Artery, pronounced LEE-ma; aka LITA, Left Internal Thoracic Artery, though most people use the term LIMA. Artery located beside the breastbone on the left side, commonly used for bypass surgery.

Lipid: group of fat and fatlike substances including steroids, fats and fatty acids.

LMWH: short for Low Molecular Weight Heparin, a form of heparin (an anti-coagulant) given to prevent blood clots. Common example is Lovenox.

Lumen: the open area inside a hollow tube, such as the lumen of an artery.

LVAD: short for Left Ventricular Assist Device, a machine which moves blood out of a severely weak left ventricle, which is usually implanted surgically. Designed to function for months, often in preparation for heart transplantation.

LVH: short for Left Ventricular Hypertrophy, a condition where the myocardial muscle cells of the left ventricle become hypertrophied, or bigger in volume. I think of it as not exactly a disease but more of a response to high demand, such as high blood pressure, which is forcing the myocardium to work more than usual.

MAZE: a form of ablation done as part of a heart operation, designed to treat atrial fibrillation.

Median sternotomy: traditional method used to access the heart and aorta, involving a cut through the breastbone from top to bottom.

MI: short for Myocardial Infarction; see Heart Attack.

MID-CAB: short for Minimally Invasive Direct Coronary Artery Bypass, a heart bypass operation utilizing a small incision of the left chest, which avoids cutting the breastbone . Usually performed Off-Pump and involves connecting the LIMA to LAD.

Mitral Prolapse: aka Mitral Valve Prolapse. Involves movement of one or both mitral valve leaflets out of the normal plane (excessive motion). May or may not cause leakage of the mitral valve and may or may not need to be fixed.

Mitral Regurgitation: abbreviated MR, aka mitral insufficiency; for some reason the term "mitral insufficiency" is not used often and "MR" is much more common. Involves leakage of blood in reverse direction back through the mitral valve into the left atrium when the left ventricle contracts.

Mitral Stenosis: condition involving stiffness and narrowing of the mitral valve where the mitral valve cannot open easily, impairing the motion of blood through it. The most common cause of mitral stenosis is rheumatic heart disease. Occasionally abbreviated MS but this can be mistaken for Multiple Sclerosis.

Mitral Valve: structure which regulates blood flow from the left atrium to the left ventricle; it opens to allow blood into the ventricle and then closes so blood will exit the ventricle through the aortic valve.

mmHg: short for millimeters of Mercury. Typical unit of measurement for blood pressure in the human body. A blood pressure of 120 mmHg would push a column of mercury 120 mm above the level of the artery.

Mortality: risk or incidence of death for a given population or condition.

MRI: short for Magnetic Resonance Imaging, technology which produces images of internal anatomy based on the differences in how tissues respond to a magnetic field. Not commonly used in association with CABG. The stainless steel wires used to secure the sternal bone after median sternotomy are safe for an MRI.

MRSA: short for Methicillin-Resistant Staph Aureus, a group of bacteria causing difficult to treat infections due to limited effectiveness of common antibiotic agents used to treat them.

MUGA scan: short for MUltiGated Acquisition scan, a so-called nuclear scan which uses a radiotracer to evaluate heart function.

Murmur: sound related to the motion of blood through a heart valve or abnormal structure. May or may not signify a disease or problem with the heart needing to be fixed.

MVr: short for Mitral Valve repair. Operation to surgically adjust a diseased mitral valve to restore normal function, keeping the patient's valve rather than cutting it out to replace it.

MVR: short for Mitral Valve Replacement. Operation to remove a diseased mitral valve and place a new valve.

Myocardial Infarction: death (necrosis) of heart muscle cells due to inadequate blood flow.

Myocardial ischemia: insufficient blood flow and oxygen delivery to an area of heart muscle.

Myocarditis: inflammation of the heart muscle.

Myocardium: aka heart muscle. Specialized involuntary muscle cells which make up the bulk of tissue of the walls of the heart and allow its pumping function.

Myxoma: a connective tissue tumor which classically arises in the left atrium of the heart. While not cancerous, a myxoma can cause a stroke if a piece of the tumor breaks off (causing an embolism) or can interfere with the function of a heart valve. Treatment is removal.

Narcotic: psychoactive compound derived from opium; in a medical sense, a medication used for pain control. Examples include morphine and codeine.

Nasal cannula: plastic tubing which delivers extra oxygen to the nostrils.

Necrosis: a form of cell death by auto-digestion, which occurs in response to severe cellular injury.

NG tube: short for NasoGastric tube, a plastic tube passing through the nose down into the stomach, usually used to drain fluid out of the stomach. Not typically needed for heart surgery patients.

Nitrate: class of medications converted to nitric oxide in the body, causing relaxation of smooth muscle and thus dilation of blood vessels. Nitroglycerin is a commonly used nitrate.

Noninvasive procedure: a test or therapy in which no instrument enters the body.

Normal Saline: fancy medical term for water with a small amount of salt in it, commonly used for IV fluid. Abbreviated as NS. The term "normal" refers to the concentration of the salt in that it is similar to the salt concentration in the blood (iso-normal); abnormal situations and abnormal patients do not require abnormal saline!

Normal Sinus Rhythm: a heart rhythm with temporal regularity, caused by electrical signals coming from a normally-functioning SA node (aka the sinus node). A NSR is regular, like a metronome.

NP: short for Nurse Practitioner, a medical professional who cares for patients independently, albeit under the general guidance of a physician.

NPO: short for Nil Per Os, meaning nothing by mouth. The patient is not allowed to eat or drink when NPO. Often patients are NPO for several hours prior to operation; thus, the stomach has time to empty prior to the patient lying flat, preventing fluid from refluxing up from the stomach into the mouth and then down into the lungs.

NSAIDs: short for Nonsteroidal Anti-Inflammatory Drugs, a class of medications which decrease pain and swelling by interfering with the action of prostaglandins. Common examples are Aspirin and Ibuprofen.

NSTEMI: short for Non-ST Elevation Myocardial Infarction, a heart attack that does not involve elevation of the ST segments of an EKG. Usually diagnosed by a rise in cardiac enzymes.

O2 Sat: short for Oxygen Saturation, the percent of hemoglobin in the blood bound to oxygen. Usually measured with a pulse oximeter, at a fingertip. The highest possible reading is 100%; normal is 95% or higher.

Obesity: medical condition characterized by accumulation of excess body fat to the point of negative health consequences. A person is considered obese if his/her BMI is >30 kg/m^2. By this metric, over 40% of adult Americans are obese, according to the Centers for Disease Control.

Occlusion: complete blockage of a blood vessel, resulting in stoppage of blood flow beyond the blockage.

Off-Pump Bypass: CABG operation performed with the heart beating, without use of the heart-lung machine (the "pump").

OPCAB: short for Off-Pump Coronary Artery Bypass, heart bypass surgery conducted without use of the heart-lung machine.

Open-heart: term used to describe surgery involving opening the chest in order to operate on the heart. The heart itself may or may not be opened, so this term is often used in an unclear way, IMO.

OR: short for Operating Room. Specialized area designed for sterile surgical procedures.

Orthopnea: fancy medical term for shortness of breath which occurs when lying down.

Orthostatic hypotension: low blood pressure which occurs upon standing and may lead to lightheadedness or passing out.

Outpatient: used to describe a test or procedure performed without admitting the patient to the hospital.

PA: short for Physician's Assistant, a medical professional trained to assist a physician, such as assisting a surgeon during an operation.

Pacemaker: medical device surgically placed beneath the skin which provides an electrical signal to the heart, causing the heart to beat at a set rate.

PACU: short for Post-Anesthesia Care Unit, commonly called recovery room. Heart surgery patients are transferred directly to the ICU from the OR and do not go to the PACU in most cases.

Palpation: examination by physical touch of the examiner's hands.

Palpitations: an awareness of the heart beat, often associated with the onset or presence of a cardiac dysrhythmia.

Paroxysmal atrial fibrillation: form of afib which is episodic, meaning it comes and goes.

PAT: short for Pre-Admission Testing, which is a set of tests performed a day or two prior to elective admission to the hospital for surgery.

Patent: pronounced PAY-tent; medical term describing a structure being open. If a stent is patent, for instance, the stent is open and blood is flowing through it.

PCI: short for Percutaneous Coronary Intervention, a procedure performed on the coronary arteries through the skin. Procedures include stent placement, atherectomy, and brachytherapy. Since atherectomy and brachytherapy are relatively uncommon, in common usage, PCI usually refers to insertion of a coronary stent.

PCP: short for Primary Care Physician, your general doctor.

PE: short for Pulmonary Embolism, a blood clot lodged in one or more of the pulmonary arteries. Often originates as a DVT in a leg vein, which moves through the right atrium and tricuspid valve and right ventricle into the pulmonary artery. Can be life-threatening if the blood clot is large and blocks the main pulmonary artery, preventing blood from leaving the right ventricle and getting into the lungs.

PEP: short for Positive Expiratory Pressure device. A plastic device – looks like a kazoo – which helps build strength of breathing after surgery.

Percutaneous: from Latin *per cutem* meaning through the skin. Refers to a medical procedure performed with puncture of the skin with a needle, rather than an open exposure by cutting the skin with a scalpel.

Pericardial effusion: an accumulation of fluid within the pericardial sac around the heart. If a pericardial effusion enlarges quickly, the pressure inside the pericardial space will increase and the heart can begin to struggle, a condition known as cardiac tamponade.

Pericardiocentesis: procedure whereby a needle is used to drain fluid from the pericardial sac.

Pericarditis: inflammation of the pericardium. When it occurs after bypass surgery, can cause more pain and prolonged soreness for the patient than is usually experienced.

Pericardium: the sac of connective tissue encasing the heart. The pericardium is thin but strong, similar to a burlap sack. A thin film of fluid lubricates the heart inside the pericardium.

PFO: short for Patent Foramen Ovale, a remnant of the foramen ovale, which is found in normal fetal development and usually closes at birth. Can be associated with rare forms of stroke but in the absence of symptoms, a PFO does not require treatment.

PFTs: short for Pulmonary Function Tests, designed to gauge a person's lung capacity. Involves blowing air out through the mouth into a machine.

Placebo: inactive substance or therapy which may possibly still have a healing or beneficial effect for a patient.

Plaque: aka atheromatous plaque. Deposits of fat, cholesterol, immune cells, calcium and other microscopic debris which accumulate on the intimal lining of arteries.

Plasma: the liquid part of the blood.

Platelets: aka thrombocytes; component of blood which reacts to blood vessel injury by clumping and initiating formation of a blood clot. Circulating platelets have no nucleus and usually last 7-8 days.

Pleural effusion: accumulation of fluid around the lung, that is, outside of the lung but within the rib cage.

Pneumothorax: abnormal collection of air outside the lung and inside the ribcage. A tension pneumothorax refers to such a collection of air with high pressure, high enough to push the heart out of normal position and be dangerous or even fatal.

POD: short for Post-Op Day, referring to a day after surgery. POD1 is the first day after surgery; most patients can expect to go home on POD4 or POD5 after heart bypass surgery.

PRN: short for Pro Re Nata, a Latin phrase meaning as the need arises. Used with medications that are taken as needed, such as most pain medicine, in contrast to scheduled medications, which are taken at a given time regardless of perceived need.

Prognosis: medical prediction of the outcome or likely result of a disease or condition.

Prophylaxis: fancy medical word for prevention.

Prostaglandin: class of lipid chemicals in the body which have hormone-like effects and play a big role in inflammation. Prostaglandins were first isolated from seminal fluid, which is produced in the prostate gland, a fact which gave the term its origin.

Protamine: a medication derived from salmon sperm which counteracts the anticoagulant effect of heparin.

Proximal: close to the center or point of attachment or origin.

PTCA: short for Percutaneous Transluminal Coronary Angioplasty, which in common parlance usually is called simply "angioplasty;" see Angioplasty.

Pulmonary: having to do with the lungs.

Pulmonary edema: abnormal accumulation of fluid in the lung tissues.

Pulmonary hypertension: elevated blood pressure within the arteries of the lungs, which creates additional mechanical work for the right ventricle.

Pulmonic valve: structure which regulates blood flow from the right ventricle to the pulmonary artery.

Pulse Ox: short for Pulse Oximeter, a medical device which estimates the oxygen saturation of hemoglobin in the red blood cells of the blood using light absorption through the skin, typically at a fingertip.

Pump head: slang term for temporary confusion occurring after heart surgery when the heart-lung machine has been used. This term is not used much anymore due to its vague meaning.

Purkinje fibers: specialized fibers in the ventricular walls which transmit electrical pulses.

PVC: short for Premature Ventricular Contraction, an "early" heartbeat which originates from Purkinje fibers in the ventricles rather than the SA node. May feel like a "skipped beat" to a patient. An occasional PVC is normal and not usually dangerous.

Radial artery: one of two arteries in the forearm providing blood to the hand. Can be used as conduit for CABG.

RBBB: short for Right Bundle Branch Block, delay or impairment of electrical signals along the right-sided pathway of the ventricular septum.

RBCs: short for Red Blood Cells, aka erythrocytes. Cells which contain hemoglobin and transport oxygen in the blood. RBCs are the most numerous cell type in the body, making up roughly 80% of all cells, some 25 trillion. Unlike most cells, RBCs do not have a nucleus.

RCA: short for Right Coronary Artery, one of the major coronary arteries, which courses on the right side of the heart.

Regurgitation: aka insufficiency.

Abnormal flow of blood in reverse direction through a heart valve. Degree of regurgitation is usually described as None, Trace, Mild, Moderate or Severe. Severe regurgitation will often cause symptoms.

Renal: fancy medical word whch means relating to the kidneys.

Resection: fancy medical word for surgical removal of tissue.

Resident: a physician who is training in a specialized field of medicine or surgery. Term came about because trainees worked so much they lived at the hospital. A resident is more senior than an intern and less experienced than a fellow.

Resolve: to go away, to become normal again.

Re-stenosis: narrowing of a blood vessel or stent which was previously opened through intervention.

RHC: short for Right Heart Catheterization, a procedure performed by interventional cardiologist to evaluate pressures within the right heart.

Rheumatic Heart Disease: inflammatory disease of the heart caused by rheumatic fever, which results from untreated Streptococcus pyogenes (ala "Strep throat"). Can cause dysfunction and scarring of heart valves years after the infection. Not seen much in the US now due to widespread use of antibiotics in treating children.

Right atrium: from Latin *atrium* "entry hall;" the heart chamber blood enters when returning from the body to the heart.

RT: short for Respiratory Therapist, a healthcare professional who specializes in providing care related to the improvement of breathing.

RVR: short for Rapid Ventricular Response; atrial fibrillation with a HR >100 beats per minute.

SA node: short for SinoAtrial node, the collection of cells in the heart that creates an electrical impulse which passes to the muscle cells causing contraction. The SA node sets the heart rate under normal conditions, influenced by the vagus nerve and sympathetic nerve fibers, as well as hormones.

Saphenous vein: one of the large veins in the leg commonly used in CABG. More specifically called the Greater Saphenous Vein.

SAVR: short for Surgical Aortic Valve Replacement, an operation involving an open incision and the heart-lung machine to replace an aortic valve, in contrast to TAVR, where a new valve is placed percutaneously.

Sclerosis: hardening of tissue.

Scrub tech: slang for surgical technologist. A medical professional trained in operating room equipment and instruments, who facilitates the steps and conduct of an operation. Vivien Thomas was a famous scrub tech who helped Dr. Alfred Blalock perform complex heart surgeries despite having only a high-school education.

Sedentary: from Latin *sedere* which means "to sit," indicating a person does not perform much physical activity.

Sepsis: a life-threatening condition related to the body's response to severe infection.

Septum: the muscular wall separating left and right chambers of the heart. The interatrial septum separates the left and right atria, while the interventricular septum separates the left and right ventricles. A PFO is a (relatively) normal defect present in the interatrial septum in ~15% of adults. There are no normal defects in the interventricular septum.

Serum: the liquid portion of the blood without the proteins involved in blood clotting.

Shock: a condition in which blood flow to body organs is inadequate. Signified by low blood pressure — often severely low — which does not improve with IV fluids.

Shunt: a tube connecting two previously unconnected parts of the body, allowing fluid to flow. Not to be confused with stent.

Sick Sinus Syndrome: a collection of complex cardiac dysrhythmias arising from dysfunction of the SA node. Often the patient will go back and forth between high heart rates and low heart rates.

Silent ischemia: episodes of impaired blood flow to myocardium which are not recognized by the patient as symptoms.

Single-vessel disease: CAD which involves only one of the coronary arteries.

Skin-to-skin: term used in surgery to describe the time from the first cut of the skin with the scalpel to the final closure of skin with suture. It is the most precise account of the duration of operative technique, whereas a patient may be in the OR longer for preparation prior to the incision and stabilization after closure.

SNF: pronounced SNIFF, short for Skilled Nursing Facility. A facility which provides nursing care.

SOB: short for Shortness of Breath.

Sodium: chemical element with symbol Na, found in table salt. Important in regulation of cellular processes.

Sonogram: synonym for ultrasound.

Spasm: sudden, involuntary contraction of muscle.

Sphygmomanometer: fancy medical term for the instrument which measures blood pressure, as in, a blood pressure cuff.

Stable angina: chest pain or discomfort which starts with exertion and stops with rest.

STAT: short for Latin *statim*, meaning immediately.

Statin: medication used to lower cholesterol levels by inhibiting the enzyme HMG-coA reductase, which is needed for the body to make cholesterol. Lovastatin was the first statin approved by the FDA, in 1987.

STEMI: short for ST-Elevation

Myocardial Infarction. A heart attack which causes changes to the ST segments on an EKG. Considered the most dangerous type of heart attack, requiring immediate therapy.

Stenosis: narrowing of an opening, such as a blood vessel or heart valve.

Stent: a tube used to keep a passageway open. A coronary stent is a metal tube used to keep a coronary artery open after balloon angioplasty.

Stent thrombosis: abrupt closure (occlusion) of a stent resulting from the formation of a blood clot.

Sternal notch: the top of the breast bone. You can feel the sternal notch as a bony V at the bottom of your neck.

Sternal wires: stainless steel wires used to bring the two halves of the breastbone back together securely after median sternotomy.

Sternotomy: See median sternotomy.

Sternum: the breastbone, in the middle front of the chest.

Stroke: damage to brain cells due to reduced blood flow and oxygen delivery. May be due to a blockage in an artery (ischemic stroke) or due to bleeding (hemorrhagic stroke).

Sublingual: method of medication absorption under the tongue, which tends to allow a fast onset of action. Nitroglycerin is often given in a sublingual form.

Supine: fancy medical term to describe lying face up.

SVC: short for Superior Vena Cava, the large vein which drains blood from the upper body (head & arms) into the right atrium of the heart.

Swan-Ganz Catheter: catheter placed percutaneously in a vein, usually in the neck, which can measure blood flow and pressure in chambers of the heart. Commonly called "the swan."

Syncope: medical term for loss of consciousness or fainting, generally due to a brief impairment of blood flow to the brain.

Systemic Circulation: the circuit blood travels in moving from the heart to the body tissues and back to the heart.

Systole: the time period during which the heart muscle contracts.

Systolic Blood Pressure: the highest blood pressure measured in the arteries, which occurs when the heart is in the contraction phase of the cardiac cycle. A common BP reading is 120/80 mmHg, where 120mmHg is the systolic pressure.

Tachycardia: a heart rate that is faster than normal; in general, a resting heart rate >100 beats per minute.

Tamponade: pronounced TAM-pon-odd, aka cardiac tamponade. A condition in which a pericardial effusion increases the pressure within the pericardial space, impairing function of the heart. Tamponade can be deadly if not promptly relieved by drainage of the pericardial effusion.

Target: the location on a coronary artery where a bypass graft is attached.

TAVR: short for Transcatheter Aortic Valve Replacement, a procedure which replaces a stenotic aortic valve without an open incision or the heart-lung machine. Often a trans-femoral approach is used, meaning access is made through the femoral artery in the groin.

TECAB: short for Totally Endoscopic Coronary Artery Bypass, a method of CABG involving use of robotic technology to both harvest conduit and complete the anastomoses.

TEE: short for Trans Esophageal Echocardiography, an imaging method which uses sound waves to generate images of the heart via a probe placed into the esophagus.

Telemetry: system used to monitor a patient's heart rate and rhythm from a remote location. The telemetry ward at a facility is often called Tele, pronounced Tell-ee.

Tension pneumothorax: a collection of air outside the lung, with increased pressure such that heart function is affected. Can be life-threatening if the air pocket is not relieved by insertion of a chest tube.

Thoracic: having to do with the chest, the thorax.

Thrill: vibration of the skin which can be felt overlying the turbulent flow of blood.

Thrombocytopenia: abnormal condition of low platelet count in the blood.

Thrombosis: formation of a blood clot within a blood vessel, obstructing blood flow through the vessel. Can occur within a stent, which would be called in-stent thrombosis.

Thrombus: a blood clot, typically meaning one located inside a blood vessel.

TIA: short for Transient Ischemic Attack, neurologic dysfunction caused by temporary impairment in blood flow, which lasts less than an hour. A TIA leaves no permanent damage to the brain, in contrast to a CVA.

tPa: short for tissue plasminogen activator, a protein naturally produced by the human body, which converts the major enzyme needed to break down blood clots. Found in endothelial cells, which line blood vessels. Manufactured as a medication given in certain cases of thrombosis, such as a STEMI where the patient cannot be promptly delivered to a cath lab.

Tricuspid valve: structure which regulates blood flow from the right atrium to the right ventricle.

Triple-vessel disease: CAD involving all three major coronary arteries. Alternatively called "3-vessel disease."

Troponin: enzyme found only in heart muscle cells which if detected in the blood indicates muscle damage and thus heart attack.

Type and Cross: short for Type and Crossmatch, a lab test/process used to determine a patient's blood type and compatibility in preparation for possible blood transfusion.

Unstable angina: chest pain or discomfort at rest, or more severe or frequent symptoms compared to previous. Unstable angina is more concerning for potential danger than stable angina.

UTI: short for Urinary Tract Infection, slang term is "bladder infection." The risk of UTI increases with the length of time a Foley catheter is kept in place.

Vagus nerve: cranial nerve X (Roman numeral ten), which is part of the autonomic nervous system, providing fibers to the heart, lungs, and digestive organs. It "wanders" throughout the torso and slows the heart rate.

Variant angina: aka Prinzmetal angina; form of chest discomfort primarily due to spasm of coronary arteries rather than atherosclerotic plaque. Unlike stable angina, the symptom pattern of variant angina tends to be unrelated to exertion.

Varicose veins: dilated veins near the surface of the legs which are engorged with blood, often due to damaged or leaking valves within the veins.

Vasectomy: surgical procedure wherein the vas deferens is cut, tied, or sealed so that sperm do not enter the urethra.

Vasoconstrictor: medication which causes smooth muscle in artery walls to contract, causing a decrease in size of the lumen.

Vasodilator: medication which causes smooth muscle in artery walls to relax, increasing the size of the lumen.

Vasopressor: medication which raises the blood pressure.

Ventilator: a machine which pushes air into the lungs through a tube in the mouth (the ET tube), to allow a patient to breathe while under an anesthetic or while otherwise unable to breathe adequately.

Ventricular fibrillation: abnormal heart rhythm characterized by disorganized contraction of myocardium, leading to impaired movement of blood out of the heart. Can be fatal if not quickly remedied by defibrillation.

Vibranium: fictional substance, strongest in the Marvel superhero universe.

VSD: short for Ventricular Septal Defect, a hole in the wall of muscle between the ventricles (interventricular septum). Could be a congenital defect or a complication of myocardial infarction. Any VSD is abnormal and in adults, a VSD usually requires closure.

Widowmaker: slang term for a heart attack involving the LAD.

Xiphoid: cartilage located at the bottom of the breastbone (sternum).

Zipper club: slang term used by heart surgery patients, referring to the scar on the mid-chest.

COMMON MEDICATIONS USED BEFORE & AFTER BYPASS SURGERY

AMIODARONE

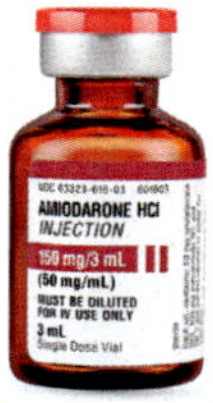

Anti-dysrhythmic ==> helps convert an abnormal heart rhythm to a normal rhythm

Used to treat afib

Given IV for 24 hours, then as a pill 1-2 times per day

Usually stopped after several weeks due to possible effects on the lungs

ASPIRIN

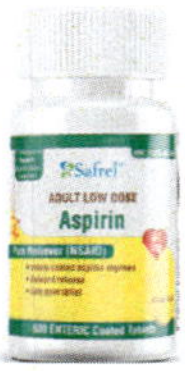

aka ACETYLSALICYLIC ACID

NSAID ==> reduces prostaglandin production, thereby decreasing inflammation & improving pain

Used to treat CAD & many other conditions

Pill taken once per day

325mg = full dose

81 mg = 'baby" dose

Can cause easy bruising & may contribute to stomach ulceration

COLACE

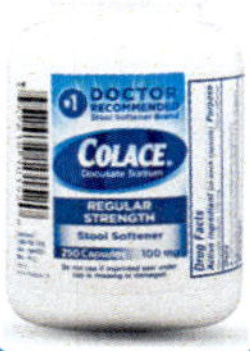

aka DOCUSATE

Stool softener ==> increases amount of water absorbed by stool in the gut, thereby making stool easier to pass

Used to treat constipation

Taken as a pill 1-3 times per day

Doesn't have many side effects but can lead to diarrhea

COUMADIN

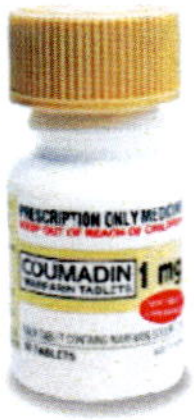

aka WARFARIN

Anti-coagulant ==> interferes with the clotting cascade of blood

Used to treat afib & mechanical heart valves

Pill taken once per day, dose varies person to person depending on metabolism

Must check a blood test known as INR, to see how "thin" the blood is

Bruising is common & severe bleeding can occur

LASIX

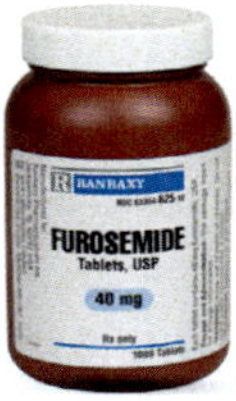

aka FUROSEMIDE

Diuretic ==> increases the production of urine

Used to treat fluid retention

Pill or IV dose taken once or twice per day

Can deplete the body of potassium so a KCl is also given

Can cause dehydration & electrolyte imbalances

LIPITOR

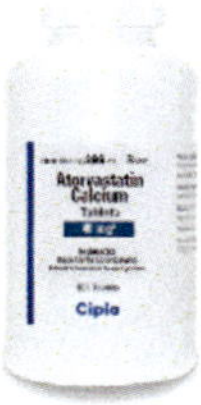

aka ATORVASTATIN

Statin ==> blocks HMGCoA-reductase, an enzyme the body uses to make cholesterol

Used treat high cholesterol & CAD

Pill taken once per day

Can cause muscle aches & headaches

LOVENOX

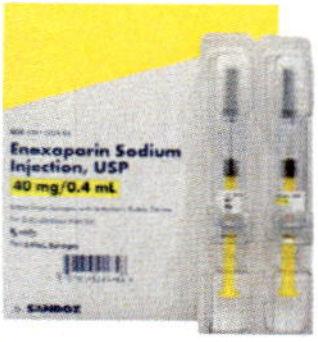

aka ENOXAPARIN

Anti-coagulant ==> interferes with the clotting cascade of blood

Low Molecular Weight form of Heparin

Used to help prevent DVTs in hospitalized patients

Given as injection under the skin, 2-3 times per day

Can cause bruising

LOPRESSOR

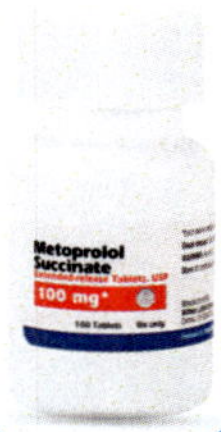

aka METOPROLOL

Beta-blocker ==> blocks the Beta receptor on smooth & cardiac muscle thereby slowing the heart rate & lowering blood pressure

Used to treat hypertension

Pill taken 1-3 times per day

Can cause dizziness, tiredness & low heart rate

MORPHINE

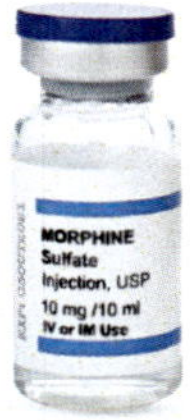

Opiate ==> analgesic pain medicine which has direct action on the central nervous system

Used to treat severe pain

Available in IV, IM, PO forms

Can cause constipation, hallucinations, central nervous system depression, death, addiction

NORCO

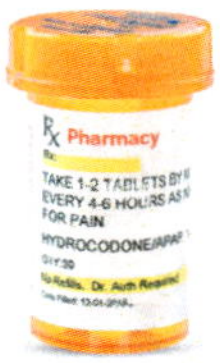

aka HYDROCODONE

- Opiate ==> analgesic pain medicine which has direct action on the central nervous system
- Has both opiate & acetaminophen components
- Used to treat moderate to severe pain
- Pill taken every few hours as needed
- Can cause constipation, hallucinations, addiction, central nervous system depression & death in large doses

PLAVIX

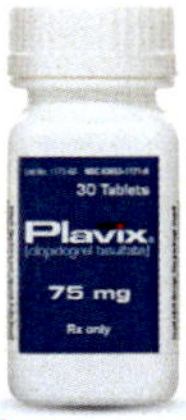

aka CLOPIDOGREL

- Antiplatelet agent ==> binds platelet receptor which decreases platelet activity & reduces risk of thrombus formation
- Used after heart attacks & placement of stents
- Pill taken once per day
- Can cause easy bruising
- Has no reversal agent — takes 7 days for effect to wear off, as new platelets form

TORADOL

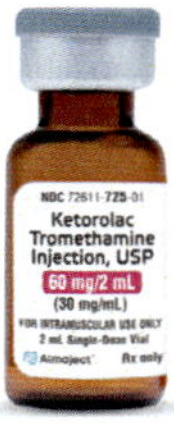

aka KETOROLAC

- NSAID ==> reduces prostaglandin production, thereby decreasing inflammation & improving pain
- More potent than Aspirin or Ibuprofen
- Used for moderate to severe pain
- Given IV every 6 hours as needed
- Can cause kidney dysfunction, so not given for >5 days

REFERENCE SOURCES

[1] https://www.who.int/health-topics/cardiovascular-diseases

[2] https://www.cdc.gov/heartdisease/facts.htm

[3] Moriyama, Iwao; *Cardiovascular Diseases in the United States*, Cambridge, 1971.

[4] Thom et al; Heart Disease and Stroke Statistics - 2006 Update: A Report from the American Heart Association Statistics Committee and Stroke Statistics Subcommittee; *Circulation*, 2006.- 113: pp 85-151.

[5] https://www.cdc.gov/nchs/covid19/mortality-overview.htm

[6] Wachowski, L., & Wachowski, L.; The Matrix Reloaded. Warner Bros, 2003.

[7] "Ashe Undergoes Bypass Surgery," *The New York Times*, Dec 14, 1979.

[8] "Artery Blocked, Letterman Has Heart Bypass Surgery," *The New York Times*, Jan 15, 2000.

[9] Cheney, Dick; *Heart: An American Medical Odyssey*, New York, 2013.

[10] "Regis Philbin Returns After Heart Surgery," *Reuters*, Apr 26, 2007.

[11] "Heart Surgery Gives Burt Reynolds 'New Pipes,'" *CNN*, Mar 3, 2010.

[12] "Local News in Brief: James Garner Has Bypass," *Los Angeles Times*, Apr 22, 1988.

[13] King, Larry; *Mr. King, You're Having a Heart Attack*, New York, 1989.

[14] "Clinton Is Given Bypass Surgery For 4 Arteries," *The New York Times*, Sept 7, 2004.

[15] "Fifty years of coronary artery bypass grafting," Ludovic Melly, et al. *J Thorac Dis* 2018 Mar; 10(3): pp 1960–1967.

[16] "Considerations Concerning the Fundaments of Theoretical Phys ics," Einstein, A.; *Science* 1940 May; 91(2369).

[17] Langer, Glenn; *Understanding Disease: How Your Heart, Lungs, Blood, and Blood Vessels Function & Respond to Treatment*, Ft. Bragg, 1999.

[18] Glynn, John; *The Story of Blood*, New York, 1948.

[19] "Determinants of kidney oxygen consumption and their relation ship to tissue oxygen tension in diabetes and hypertension," Hansell, Peter, et al. *Clin Exp Pharmacol Physiol* 2013 Feb; 40(2): pp 123–137.

[20] Neuhof, Selian; *The Heart: Its Physiology, Pathology and Clinical Aspects*, Philadelphia, 1923.

[21] "Hooked on heart regeneration: the zebrafish guide to recovery," Stewart K., et al. *Cardiovascular Research* 2022 May; 118(7): pp 1667-1679.

[22] Gibson, George; *Diseases of the Heart and Aorta*, London, 1898.

[23] Snellen, H.A.; *History of Cardiology*, Rotterdam, 1984.

[24] Norman, John; *Coronary Artery Medicine and Surgery*, London, 1975.

[25] Gould, Sylvester; *Pathology of the Heart and Blood Vessels*, Springfield, 1968.

[26] "Tennis Courts in the Human Body: A Review of the Misleading Metaphor in Medical Literature," Rao, A. *Cureus* 2022 Jan; 14(1).

[27] Fishman, Alfred; *Circulation of the Blood: Men and Ideas*, American Physiological Society, New York, 1982.

[28] Haggard, Howard; *The Doctor in History*, New Haven, 1934.

[29] Bynum, W.F., et al; *The Emergence of Modern Cardiology*, London, 1985.

[30] Hirschfelder, Arthur; *Diseases of the Heart and Aorta*, 3rd ed., Phil adelphia, 1918.

[31] "Naming of the Waves in the EKG, with a Brief Account of their Genesis," Hurst, J.; *Circulation* 1998 Nov; 98: pp 1937-1942.

[32] "Heroin & Aspirin The Connection & The Collection - Part I," Mun sey, C.; *Bottles and Extras* 2007 Jan.

[33] "The human coronary collateral circulation: development and clinical importance," Seiler, C.; *European Heart Journal* 2013 Sept; 34(34).

[34] "A Review of the Impella Devices," Zein, R.; *Interventional Cardiology* 2022 Apr 17(5).

[35] Frink, Richard; *Inflammatory Atherosclerosis: Characteristics of the Injurious Agent*, Sacramento, 2002.

[36] Hobbie, Russell; *Intermediate Physics for Medicine and Biology*, 3rd ed., New York, 1997.

[37] Altschule, Mark; *Physiology in Disease of the Heart and Lungs*, Cambridge, 1949.

[38] Rolleston, Humphrey; *The Harveian Oration*, Cambridge, 1928.

[39] Cabot, Blake; *The Motion of the Heart*, New York, 1954.

[40] Haeger, Kurt; *The Illustrated History of Surgery*, Gothenburg, 2000.

[41] Singh, Bramah; *Silent Myocardial Ischemia and Angina*, New York, 1988.

[42] "The Utility of Gestures in Patients with Chest Discomfort," Marcus, G., et al; *Am Journ Med* 2007 Jan; 120(1).

[43] "Cardiac chest pain: does body language help the diagnosis?" Edmondstone, W.; *Br Med J* 1995 Dec; 311.

[44] Rapaport, Elliot; *Cardiology and Co-Existing Disease*, New York, 1994.

[45] Plotz, Milton; *Coronary Heart Disease*, London, 1957.

[46] Gregg, Donald.; *Coronary Circulation in Health and Disease*, Philadelphia, 1950.

[47] www.fda.gov

[48] "Carbon Monoxide Poisoning," Blumenthal, I.; *Journal of the Royal Society of Medicine* 2001 Jun; 94(6).

[49] *Texas Heart Institute Heart Owner's Handbook*, New York, 1996.

[50] Fuster, Valentin, et al; *Atherosclerosis and Coronary Artery Disease* Volume 1, Philadelphia, 1996.

[51] Conn, Hadley; *Cardiac and Vascular Diseases*, Vol II, London, 1971.

[52] "2018 AHA/ACC/AACVPR/AAPA/ABC/ACPM/ADA/AGS/APhA/ASPC/NLA/PCNA Guideline on the Management of Blood Choles terol: A Report of the American College of Cardiology/American Heart Association Task Force on Clinical Practice Guidelines," Grundy, S., et al; *Circulation* 2018 Nov; 139 (25).

[53] "Dietary cholesterol, heart disease risk and cognitive dissonance," McNamara, D.; *Proc Nutr Soc* 2014 May; 73(2).

[54] "Dietary cholesterol and the risk of cardiovascular disease in patients: a review of the Harvard Egg Study and other data," Jones, P.; *Int J Clin Pract Suppl* 2009 Oct; 163.

[55] https://www.cdc.gov/genomics/disease/fh/FH.htm

[56] "Genetics of Coronary Disease," McPherson, R.; *Circulation Research* 2016 Feb; 118(4).

[57] "Exercise and Cardiovascular Health," Myers, J.; *Circulation* 2003 Jan; 107(1).

[58] Cooper, Kenneth; *Aerobics*, New York, 1968.

[59] Cooper, Kenneth; *It's Better to Believe: The New Medical Program That Uses Spiritual Motivation To Achieve Maximum Health And Add Years To Your Life*, Nashville, 1995.

[60] "Coronary artery bypass surgery in elderly people," Natarajan, A., et al; *Postgrad Med J.* 2007 Mar; 83(977): pp 154–158.

[61] "Provisional Life Expectancy Estimates for January through June, 2020," Arias, E., et al; *U.S. Department of Health and Human Services National Vital Statistics System Vital Statistics Rapid Re lease* 2021 Feb; 010.

[62] "Role of personality in cardiovascular diseases: An issue that needs to be focused too!" Sahoo, S.; *Indian Heart J* 2018 Dec; 70 (3).

[63] "Sleep Duration as a Risk Factor for Cardiovascular Disease- a Review of the Recent Literature," Nagai, M.; *Curr Cardiol Rev* 2010 Feb; 6(1).

[64] "Obesity in Coronary Heart Disease: An Unaddressed Behavioral Risk Factor," Ades, P.; *Prev Med* 2017 Nov; 104.

[65] "Association of Habitual Alcohol Intake With Risk of Cardiovascular Dis ease," Biddinger, K., et al; *JAMA Network Open* 2022 Mar.

[66] "Evidence for a Direct Harmful Effect of Alcohol on Myocardial Health: A Large Cross-Sectional Study of Consumption Patterns and Cardiovascular Disease Risk Biomarkers From Northwest Rus sia, 2015 to 2017," Iankunchykova, O., et al; *J Am Heart Assoc* 2020 Jan; 9 (1).

[67] "Infections, Inflammation, and the Risk of Coronary Heart Disease," Roivaineon, M., et al; *Circulation* 2000 Jan; 101(3).

[68] Clear, James; *Atomic Habits*, New York, 2018.

[69] Murphy, Joseph; *The Power of Your Subconscious Mind: Unlock Your Master Key to Success*, Radford, 2007.

[70] Lee, Shannon; *Be Water, My Friend: The Teachings of Bruce Lee*, Ebury Publishing, 2020.

[71] "Hyperdynamic Left Ventricular Function: Good or Bad News?" Crawford, M.; *Clin Card Alert* 2020 May.

[72] "Werner Forssmann Nobel Prize for physiology or medicine 1956: Mark Nicholls looks at the courageous role Werner Forssmann played in the development of cardiac catheterization and the subsequent award of the 1956 Nobel Prize for his endeavours," Nicholls, Mark; *European Heart J* 2020 Mar; 41 pp 980-982.

[73] "A Half Century of Selective Coronary Arteriography," Bruschke, A., et al; *J Am College Card* 2009 Dec; 54 (23).

[74] "Balloon Angioplasty – The Legacy of Andreas Grüntzig, M.D. (1939–1985)," Barton, M., et al; *Front Cardiovasc Med* 2014 Dec; 29(1).

[75] Cameron, John; *Physics of the Body*, 2017.

[76] "Stent; The Man and Word Behind the Coronary Metal Prosthesis," Roguin, A; *Circulation: Cardiovascular Interventions* 2011 Apr; 4: pp 206-209.

[77] "Stent thrombosis: definitions, mechanisms and prevention," Grove, E.; *e-Euro Soc Card* 2007 May; 5(32).

[78] "Aspirin Use to Prevent Cardiovascular Disease: US Preventive Services Task Force Recommendation Statement," *JAMA* 2022 Apr; 327(16).

[79] Bourne, Geoffrey, *Hearts and Heart-like Organs*, Vol 3, New York, 1980.

[80] "Anatomic variations and anomalies of the coronary arteries: 64-slice CT angiographic appearance," Kosar, P., et al; *Diag Interv Radiol* 2009 Dec; 15(4).

[81] Mick Jagger and Keith Richards; You Can't Always Get What You Want, Let It Bleed album 1969.

[82] "Do Hospitals and Surgeons With Higher Coronary Artery Bypass Graft Surgery Volumes Still Have Lower Risk-Adjusted Mortality Rates?" Hannan, E., et al; *Circulation* 2003 Jul; 108(7).

[83] Miller, Stephen, et al; *Cardiac Imaging*, 3rd ed., Boston, 2009.

[84] "Why is the mammary artery so special and what protects it from atherosclerosis?" Otsuka, F., et al; *Annals of Cardiothoracic Sur gery* 2013 July; 2(4).

[85] "Internal mammary artery harvesting in cardiac surgery: An often mistold story," de la Cruz, Y., et al; *CorSalud* 2020 Jan-Mar; 12(1): pp 64-76.

[86] "Alexis Carrel's historic leap of faith," Levin, S.; *Historical Vignettes in Vascular Surgery* 2015 Mar; 61(3): pp 832-833.

[87] "The Discovery of Heparin," McLean, J.; *Circulation* 1959 Jan; 19(1).

[88] "From Farm to Pharma: An Overview of Industrial Heparin Manufacturing Methods," van der Meer, J., et al; *Molecules* 2017 Jun; 22(6).

[89] "Evolution of Cardiopulmonary Bypass," Stoney, W.; *Circulation* 2009 Jan; 119(21).

[90] "Review article: Heparin and protamine during cardiac surgery," Aren, C.; *Perfusion* 1989 July 4(3).

[91] Senders, John; *Human Error: Cause, Prediction, and Reduction*, New York, 1991.

[92] "Postoperative atrial fibrillation following cardiac surgery: a persistent complication," Greenberg, J., et al; *Euro J CardioThor Surg* 2017 Oct; 52(4).

[93] https://health.ucsd.edu/for-health-care-professionals/anticoagula tion-guidelines/warfarin

[94] "Rate Control versus Rhythm Control for Atrial Fibrillation after Cardiac Surgery," Gillinov, M., et al; *NEJM* 2016 May; 374.

[95] "Trends in use of off-pump coronary artery bypass grafting: Results from the Society of Thoracic Surgeons Adult Cardiac Surgery Database," Ba kaeen, F., et al; *J Thoracic & Cardiovascular Surgery* 2014 Jan; 148(3).

[96] https://www.goodreads.com/quotes.

APPRECIATION

Thank you, Jessica, for your love and support. You are the most amazing person I know.

Thank you, John Mark, for helping me write and re-write this book, and providing encouragement at every step. You are not only my son but my close friend.

Thank you, JJ, for your encouragement and your editorial insights. You inspire me with your selfless ambition to do God's work.

Thank you, Mom, for reviewing my manuscript and your relentless encouragement and prayers, not just for this book but for my entire life. Dad, thank you for modeling for me a life of hard work and contented faith.

Thank you, Dana King, for your keen eye for grammar and your valued suggestions. Mason, thank you for being a great friend — and my faithful personality coach!

Thank you, Mo Safi, for your artistic skill and design genius — and your diligent hard work. Thank you for not giving up on me!

Thank you, Dr. Kon and Dr. Kincaid, for teaching me how to operate with excellence and how to care for heart patients. Dr. Shires, thank you for teaching me that complex surgeries are just simple steps performed in the correct order and how to talk so patients can understand.

Thank you, all of my patients, for trusting me and allowing me the privilege of caring for you.

Thank you, Lord, for the strength for today. And bright hope for tomorrow. Hope built on the love of Jesus Christ.

J. Mark Pool

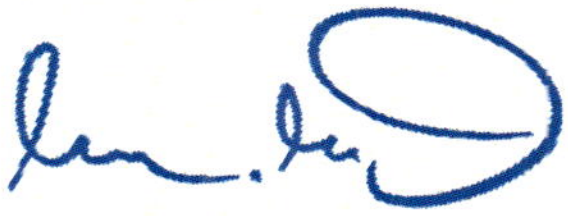

Made in United States
Orlando, FL
08 January 2025

57033289R00113